# SAFE TRANSFER AND RETRIEVAL

# SAFE TRANSFER AND RETRIEVAL

## The Practical Approach

*Advanced Life Support Group*

Edited by
Peter Driscoll
Ian Macartney
Kevin Mackway-Jones
Peter Oakley

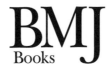

First published in 2002
by BMJ Books, BMA House, Tavistock Square,
London WC1H 9JR

www.bmjbooks.com

**British Library Cataloguing in Publication Data**

A catalogue record for this book is available from the British Library

ISBN 0 7279 1583 5

Typeset by Newgen Imaging Systems (P) Ltd., Chennai, India
Printed and bound in Spain by GraphyCems, Navarra

# CONTENTS

# WORKING GROUP

| | |
|---|---|
| **Paul Allsop** | Anaesthetics, Burton-upon-Trent |
| **Paul Baines** | Paediatric ICU, Liverpool |
| **Ruth Buckley** | Emergency Nursing, Stoke on Trent |
| **John Burnside** | Ambulance Service, Manchester |
| **Peter Driscoll** | Emergency Medicine, Manchester |
| **Mark Forrest** | ICU, Liverpool |
| **Pauline Holt** | Paediatric ICU Nursing, Liverpool |
| **Ian Macartney** | ICU, Manchester |
| **Kevin Mackway-Jones** | Emergency Medicine, Manchester |
| **Giles Morgan** | ICU, Truro |
| **Peter Oakley** | Anaesthesia/Trauma, Stoke on Trent |
| **Claire O'Connor** | ICBIS Study, Manchester |
| **Vincent O'Keeffe** | ICU, Glan Clwyd |
| **Shirley Remington** | ICU, Manchester |
| **Stephen Shaw** | ICU, Liverpool |
| **Sarah Wheatly** | Anaesthesia, Manchester |
| **Susan Wieteska** | ALSG, Manchester |

# CONTRIBUTORS

| | |
|---|---|
| **Paul Allsop** | Anaesthetics, Burton-upon-Trent |
| **Paul Baines** | Paediatric ICU, Liverpool |
| **Danielle Bryden** | Anaesthesia, Manchester |
| **Ruth Buckley** | Emergency Nursing, Stoke on Trent |
| **John Burnside** | Ambulance Service, Manchester |
| **Peter Driscoll** | Emergency Medicine, Manchester |
| **Mark Forrest** | ICU, Liverpool |
| **Tim Graham** | Cardiothoracic Surgery, Birmingham |
| **Carl Gwinnutt** | Anaesthesia, Manchester |
| **Pauline Holt** | Paediatric ICU Nursing, Liverpool |
| **Jonathan Hyde** | Cardiothoracic Surgery, West Midlands |
| **Ian Macartney** | ICU, Manchester |
| **Kevin Mackway-Jones** | Emergency Medicine, Manchester |
| **Giles Morgan** | ICU, Truro |
| **Peter Oakley** | Anaesthesia/Trauma, Stoke on Trent |
| **Claire O'Connor** | *Formerly* ICBIS Study, Manchester |
| **Vincent O'Keeffe** | ICU, Glan Clwyd |
| **Kate Olney** | ICBIS Study, Manchester |
| **Shirley Remington** | ICU, Manchester |

CONTRIBUTORS

**Stephen Shaw**                                          ICU, Liverpool

**Terence Wardle**                                     Medicine, Chester

**Sarah Wheatly**                              Anaesthesia, Manchester

**Susan Wieteska**                                  ALSG, Manchester

# PREFACE

The number of interhospital transfers continues to rise. This increasing demand for intensive care beds is fuelled by patients' and relatives' expectations and improved resuscitation and surgical techniques.

This book (and the associated course) has been developed to try to overcome the difficulties faced by healthcare professionals organising and carrying out the transportation of critically ill or injured patients. It addresses all the elements involved in transfer and provides a systematic approach.

*Safe Transfer and Retrieval: The Practical Approach* has been developed by a multiprofessional group from across the UK. It is the core text for the STaR course, but will be useful to medical and allied personnel whether they attend the course or not. The aim is to provide a systematic approach to the transfer or retrieval of a patient.

The book is divided into five parts. Part I introduces the subject by discussing the principles of the STaR approach. Part II deals with the management of the transfer or retrieval according to the principles. Part III describes the practical procedures necessary while Part IV provides an overview of the clinical care required during the assessment and stabilisation phases of the transfer. Situations requiring specific changes in the core approach are also discussed here. The appendices in Part V consider the legal and safety aspects of transfers, as well as the specific differences in helicopter transfers.

# ACKNOWLEDGEMENTS

A great many people have put a lot of hard work into the production of this book and the accompanying course. The editors would like to thank all the contributors for their efforts and all the STaR providers and instructors who took the time to send their comments during the development of the text and course.

We are greatly indebted to Helen Carruthers MMAA for producing the excellent line drawings that illustrate the text.

Finally, we would like to thank, in advance, those of you who will attend the Safe Transfer and Retrieval (STaR) course; no doubt you will have much constructive criticism to offer.

# CONTACT DETAILS AND WEBSITE INFORMATION

ALSG: www.alsg.org
Best bets: www.bestbets.org

For details on ALSG courses visit the website or contact:

Advanced Life Support Group
Second Floor, The Dock Office
Trafford Road
Salford Quays
Manchester M5 2XB
UK

Tel: +44 (0) 161 877 1999
Fax: +44 (0) 161 877 1666

Email: enquiries@alsg.org

# PART

# I

# INTRODUCTION

# 1

# Introduction

---

**Objectives**

- Understand why critically ill patients are transferred between hospitals.
- Understand the technical problems which may adversely affect patient care.

---

The STaR manual with its associated course is aimed at a multidisciplinary audience and has been developed in an attempt to overcome the difficulties faced by healthcare professionals when organising and carrying out the transportation of critically ill or injured patients. There are essentially two components:

- the organisational and management strategy
- the practical problems that may be encountered during preparation, packaging, and transportation of patients.

Although the course focus is on transportation of patients between hospitals, the same approach can be applied to the transportation of critically ill patients within hospitals.

The usual purpose of interhospital transfer or retrieval is to allow the patient to be treated more effectively in a geographically separate site. Transfer *per se* does not constitute therapy and is not without risk. It is therefore essential to consider the risk versus the benefits before undertaking a potentially hazardous journey.

In 60% of cases, the transfer results from the lack of a functioning ICU bed in the primary hospital. This could be either no bed or no nursing staff to look after the patient. The second most common cause (27·5%) is the requirement for specialist management in a tertiary centre.

Box 1.1 demonstrates the wide spectrum of clinical pathologies which may be encountered.

**Box 1.1.   Primary diagnosis in transferred patients**

Trauma (including head injuries)
Respiratory failure/pneumonia
Postoperative/surgical
Intracranial bleeds/subarachnoids
Postcardiac/respiratory arrest
Overdose
Renal failure
Multiorgan failure/sepsis
Liver failure
Pancreatitis
Burns
Aortic aneurysm
Cardiac failure
Others:
    asthma
    neurological condition
    status epilepticus
    meningitis
    diabetes
    cancer
    eclampsia

*Source*: Intensive Care Bed Information Service (ICBIS)

The source of these patients also varies widely (Box 1.2). Emergency departments and ICUs are the most frequent starting places for the movement of intensive care patients. Though it is to be expected that patients moving from an ICU will be fully stabilised and packaged, the same assumption cannot be made when patients are moved from other departments. These patients and those coming from wards and theatres may require considerable time before they are adequately prepared and packaged for transfer.

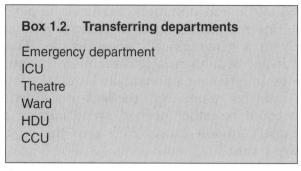

**Box 1.2.   Transferring departments**

Emergency department
ICU
Theatre
Ward
HDU
CCU

*Source*: Intensive Care Bed Information Service (ICBIS)

Transfers are not infrequently associated with adverse events, which may be recorded on transfer forms. Those seen most commonly are shown in Box 1.3.

**Box 1.3.   Adverse events**

No capnography available (when clinically indicated)
Hospital equipment failure
Significant hypotension
Significant hypoxia
Inadequate resuscitation
Significant tachycardia
Mechanical ventilator not available
Delay in getting ambulance
Ambulance getting lost en route
Cardiac arrest in ambulance

*Source*: Intensive Care Bed Information Service (ICBIS)

The number of interhospital transfers continues to rise. This increasing demand for intensive care beds is fuelled by patients' and relatives' expectations and improved resuscitation and surgical techniques.

This manual has been developed to try to overcome the difficulties faced by healthcare professionals organising and carrying out the transportation of critically ill or injured patients. It addresses all the elements involved in transfer and provides a systematic approach.

# 2

# STaR principles

**Objectives**

- Provide an overview of the principles of the safe transfer or retrieval of critically ill patients.
- Describe the systematic ACCEPT approach for managing such patients.

## INTRODUCTION

The aim of a safe transfer policy is to ensure that patient care is streamlined, and of the highest standard. To achieve this, the **right** patient has to be taken at the **right** time, by the **right** people, to the **right** place by the **right** form of transport and receive the **right** care throughout. This requires a systematic approach which incorporates a high level of planning and preparation prior to the patient being moved. One such approach is the ACCEPT method (Box 2.1).

---

**Box 2.1. The systematic approach to patient transfer**

A – assessment
C – control
C – communication
E – evaluation
P – preparation and packaging
T – transportation

---

Following ACCEPT ensures that assessments and procedures are carried out in the right order. This method also correctly emphasises the preparation that is required before the patient is transported. The component parts of ACCEPT are outlined below. Subsequent chapters deal with each part in detail.

# ASSESSMENT

The first thing to do is assess the situation. Sometimes the clinician involved in the transportation has also been involved in the care given up to that point. Commonly, however, the transporter will have been brought in specifically for that purpose and will have no prior knowledge of the patient's clinical history.

# CONTROL

Once assessment is complete, the transport organiser needs to take control of the situation. This requires:

- identification of the clinical team leader
- identification of the tasks to be carried out
- allocation of tasks to individuals or teams.

The lines of responsibility must be established urgently. In theory, ultimate responsibility is held jointly by the referring consultant clinician, the receiving consultant clinician and the transfer personnel at different stages of the transfer process. There should always be a named person with overall responsibility for organising the transfer.

# COMMUNICATION

Moving ill patients from one place to another obviously requires cooperation and the involvement of several people. Therefore key personnel need to be informed when transportation is being considered (Box 2.2).

---

**Box 2.2.   People who need to know about a transfer**

- The consultant responsible for current clinical care
- The consultant responsible for the transfer of the patient (if different from above)
- The consultant(s) responsible for intensive care
- The patient's relatives
- The consultant(s) responsible for care in the receiving unit
- Ambulance control or special transportation controls (when appropriate)

---

Communication may take a long time to complete if one person does it all. It is therefore advisable to share the tasks between appropriate people, taking into account expertise and the local policies. In all cases it is important that information is passed on clearly and unambiguously. This is particularly the case when talking to people over the telephone. It is useful to plan what to say before telephoning and to use the systematic summary shown in Box 2.3.

---

**Box 2.3.   Key elements in any communication**

- Who you are
- What is needed (from the listener)
- What are the (relevant) patient details
- What the problem is
- What has been done to address the problem
- What happened

---

The second question can be repeated at the end to help summarise the situation. The response to all these questions should be documented in the patient's notes. The person in overall charge can then assimilate this information so that a proper evaluation of the patient's requirements for transportation can be made.

## EVALUATION

The dual aims of evaluation are to assess whether transfer is appropriate for the patient and, if so, what clinical urgency the patient has. While evaluation is a dynamic process which starts from first contact with the patient it is only when the first phase of ACCEPT (that is, ACC) has been completed that enough information will have been gathered.

### Is transfer appropriate for this patient?

Critically ill patients require transfer because of the need for:

- specialist treatment
- specialist investigations unavailable in the referring hospital
- specialist facilities unavailable in the referring hospital.

The risks involved in transfer must be balanced against the risks of staying and the benefits of care that can only be given by the receiving unit.

### What clinical urgency does this patient have?

Once it has been established that transfer is needed then the urgency must be evaluated. The degree of urgency for transfer and the severity of illness may be used to rank the patient's transfer needs (see Box 2.4). This hierarchy also helps determine both the personnel required and the mode of transport.

---

**Box 2.4. Transfer categories**

- Intensive
- Time critical
- Ill and unstable
- Ill and stable
- Unwell
- Well

---

## PREPARATION AND PACKAGING

Preparation and packaging both have the aim of ensuring that the patient transport proceeds with the minimum change in level of care provided and with no deterioration in the patient's condition. The first stage (preparation) involves completion of patient stabilisation and preparation of transfer team personnel and equipment. The second stage (packaging) involves the final measures that need to be taken to ensure the security and safety of the patient during the transportation itself.

## Patient preparation

To reduce complications during any journey, meticulous resuscitation and stabilisation should be carried out prior to transfer. This may involve carrying out procedures requested by the receiving hospital or unit. The standard Airway, Breathing, and Circulation (ABC) approach is useful. The airway must be cleared and secured. Appropriate respiratory support must be established.

Venous access is essential and preferably should include a minimum of two large bore cannulae. The patient must have received adequate fluid resuscitation to ensure optimal tissue oxygenation. Hypovolaemic patients tolerate the inertial forces of transportation very poorly.

> Inadequate resuscitation or missed illnesses and injuries will result in instability during transfer and will adversely affect outcome.

## Equipment preparation

All equipment must be functioning and supplies of drugs and fluids should be more than adequate for the whole of the intended journey.

Particular care should be taken with supplies of oxygen, inotropes, sedative drugs, and batteries for portable electronic equipment.

Specialist equipment may also be required for particular patients – for example, children and those patients with spinal injuries.

A member of the team should be allocated the task of ensuring that all the patient's documents, including case notes, investigations, reports and a transfer form, accompany the patient.

The team requires a phone and contact names and numbers to enable direct communication with both the receiving and base units. In addition, all personnel need appropriate clothing, food if the journey is long, and enough money to enable them to get home if needed.

## Personnel preparation

The number and nature of staff accompanying patients during transport will reflect their transfer category.

All staff must practise within their areas of competence. For an intensive care transfer, the Intensive Care Society (ICS) recommends that the accompanying physician "should have received training in intensive care and transport medicine, had involvement in previous transfers and preferably have at least 2 years' experience in anaesthesia, intensive care medicine or other equivalent speciality". In addition, they should be accompanied by another experienced doctor, nurse, paramedic or technician familiar with intensive care procedures and with all transport equipment.

Whatever the category of the patient, all personnel should be competent in the transfer procedure and familiar with the equipment which is to be used as well as the details of the patient's clinical condition. The team should carry accident insurance with adequate provision for personal injury or death sustained during the transfer.

## Packaging

All lines and drains should be secured to the patient, the patient should be secured to the trolley, and the trolley must be secured to the ambulance.

Chest drains should be secured and unclamped with any underwater seal device replaced by an appropriate commercial drainage valve and bag system. If the patient has a simple pneumothorax or is at risk of developing one, a chest drain needs to be inserted prophylactically.

Mummy wrapping the patient provides additional security and reduces heat loss.

# TRANSPORTATION

## Mode of transport

The choice of transport needs to take into account several factors (Box 2.5).

> **Box 2.5. Factors affecting mode of transfer**
>
> - Nature of illness
> - Urgency of transfer
> - Mobilisation time
> - Geographical factors
> - Weather
> - Traffic conditions
> - Cost

Road ambulances are by far the most common means used in the United Kingdom. They have a low overall cost, rapid mobilisation time and are less affected by weather conditions. They also give rise to less physiological disturbance.

Air transfer may be used for journeys over 50 miles or two hours in duration or if road access is difficult. The speed of the journey itself has to be balanced against organisational delays and also the need for intervehicle transfer at the beginning and end of the journey.

## Care during transport

Physiological problems which occur during transportation may arise from the effects of the transport environment on the deranged physiology of the patient. Careful preparation can minimise the deleterious effects of inertial forces, such as tipping, acceleration, and deceleration, as well as changes in temperature and barometric pressure changes.

The standard of care and the level of monitoring carried out prior to transfer need to be continued, as far as possible, during the transfer. Monitoring will include oxygen saturation, ECG, and direct arterial pressure monitoring in all patients. End-tidal carbon dioxide ($CO_2$) monitoring should be used in all intubated patients.

The patient should be well covered and kept warm during the transfer. Road speed decisions depend both on clinical urgency and the availability of limited resources such as oxygen.

With adequate preparation, the transportation phase is usually incident free. However, untoward events do occur. Should this be the case, the patient needs to be reassessed using the ABC approach (see Chapter 11). Appropriate corrective measures should then be instituted. This may require a stop at the first available place. Following any untoward events, communications with the receiving unit are important. This should follow the systematic summary described previously.

## Handover

At the end of the transfer direct contact with the receiving team must be established, so that a succinct, systematic summary of the patient can then be provided. This needs to be accompanied by a written record of the patient's history, vital signs, therapy, and significant clinical events during transfer. All the other documents which have been taken with the patient should also be handed over. Whilst this is going on, the rest of the transferring team can help in moving the patient from the ambulance trolley to the receiving unit's bed. The team can then retrieve all their equipment and personnel and make their way back to their home unit.

**Summary**

The safe transfer and retrieval of a patient requires a systematic approach. The ACCEPT method ensures that important activities will be carried out at the appropriate time.

# II

# MANAGING THE
# TRANSFER – ACCEPT

# 3

# Assessment and control

**Objectives**

- Describe a systematic approach to assessing a potential transfer situation.
- Describe the steps necessary to control the situation.

## INTRODUCTION

A clinician involved in a potential transfer situation may have had no patient contact before he receives a phone call from a member of the treating clinical team. It is important to learn how to assess such a situation quickly and effectively. This must be done before patient management continues.

## ASSESSING THE SITUATION

Proper assessment requires careful consideration of both the patient's condition and the actions and capabilities of the transferring team. The answers to several key questions will help this process.

**Box 3.1.  Assessment questions**

- What is the problem?
- What is being done?
- What effect is it having?
- What is needed now?

It is also essential to find out who holds responsibility for the patient's care both now and during pretransfer treatment and during any eventual transport. In the latter case, this will usually be shared. It is preferable for named consultants in both referring and receiving units to be actively involved in any transportation decisions.

# CONTROLLING THE SITUATION

Following the initial assessment, the transfer team leader needs to take control of the situation. This involves:

- identifying the team leader
- identifying the tasks to be carried out
- allocation of tasks to individuals or teams.

## Identifying the team leader

The transfer team leader will be in overall control of the transfer; that is, they will have responsibility for organising resources and timings, ensuring communication is optimal, carrying out the evaluation, overseeing packaging, and initiating the transfer itself. They may or may not be in charge of the clinical care of the patient. If they are not then close liaison with the clinical team leader is essential.

As well as being present, the transfer team leader must be experienced enough in transfers to be capable of successfully seeing the task through and must be senior enough to have the confidence of their peers. In any given situation, an appropriate leader is usually obvious, because of either their experience or seniority. If this is not the case the most experienced member of staff present should take this role initially. More senior or experienced help should be sought urgently if this is required.

## Task identification

Transfer task identification will be greatly helped if the ACCEPT approach is used.

Once control is established then communication becomes a priority. Calls for both information and action will be needed urgently. This is discussed in more detail in Chapter 4.

Evaluation will require accurate information. A quick review of the information available versus that needed will allow areas of uncertainty to be identified.

Preparation and packaging will require equipment to be made available and staff for the transfer itself to be identified.

Clinical care must run in tandem with transfer tasks.

## Task allocation

Tasks should be allocated by the transfer team leader. Competence is the key attribute and tasks should only be given to staff who have the appropriate training and expertise. The team leader will need to consider the relative priority of each task and the scope for concurrent activity.

**Summary**

The first step of the transferring clinician is to assess the situation and determine what else the patient requires. To carry this out the doctor needs to take control of the situation by allocating key roles to staff.

# 4

# Communication

**Objectives**

- Understand who should communicate and who should be communicated with during the transfer process.
- Understand what needs to be communicated during the transfer process.

## INTRODUCTION

As has already been stated in Chapter 2, the successful transfer of an ill patient from one clinical area to another requires the coordinated effort of many individuals from a number of different teams. Good communication is essential to achieve the cooperation and coordination of these people.

Communication actually begins, on an individual level, as soon as the initial referral is received. The responsible clinician must communicate effectively with those who are already dealing with the patient so that an accurate **assessment** can be carried out. Good communication must then be continued through the **control** phase to the point when the decision to transfer has been made. At this point the agreed need for transfer must be communicated to those who need to know. The receiving clinical area must be identified and having agreed to accept the patient, the transport itself must be organised.

It is for this reason that **communication** is placed in a pivotal position on the ACCEPT approach.

Once the transfer is underway good communication remains an essential part of the process. Both dispatching and receiving teams must be kept informed, as must the transport providers. Relatives and supporting services should be kept up to date at all stages of the transfer and written records must be kept.

Many different methods of communication may be necessary during the transfer. Initially (at the dispatching unit) most will be face to face or by phone. Once transport is underway cellular phones and radios may be used. Finally, face to face communication with the receiving team will be important, as will the delivery of an accurate written record.

## WHO COMMUNICATES WITH WHOM?

The clinician responsible for the decision to transfer the patient has the ultimate responsibility for any communication that occurs both within the dispatching unit and also between this unit and outside agencies. Similarly, the accepting clinician in the receiving unit has ultimate responsibility for communication at that end of the transfer chain. Both these clinicians may have to delegate some of these calls to other members of staff. However, key calls, such as those offering and accepting the patient, should be between these two. A list of some of the calls that may be necessary during the transfer process is given below together with a list of appropriate staff who could be asked to make them.

**Table 4.1. Calls during transfer**

|  | Nature | Responsibility |
|---|---|---|
| Transfer calls | Seek availability of bed | Nurse |
|  | Book transfer | Nurse |
|  | Advise receiving unit | Nurse |
|  | Arrange staff: |  |
|  | nursing | Senior nurse |
|  | paramedical | Senior nurse |
|  | medical | Responsible clinician |
| Clinical calls | Discuss with specialist | Responsible clinician |
|  | Negotiate bed | Responsible clinician |
| Information calls | Inform responsible consultants | Junior doctor from team |
|  | Inform relatives | Senior nurse |

Even if calls are delegated, it is important that the outcome is reported to the responsible clinicians at each unit so that they maintain an overview of the transfer as it occurs.

## WHAT NEEDS TO BE COMMUNICATED?

Successful communication has occurred when all the necessary information has been passed and understood by all the relevant people. During the transfer process, successful communication can be seen to require that both clinical and transportation arrangements are made and understood. As already noted in Chapter 2, each communication should consist of:

- who you are
- what is needed (from the listener)
- what are the (relevant) patient details
- what the problem is
- what has been done to address the problem
- what happened.

## Who you are

Not only should the instigator of the call identify who they are, they should also state whether they are calling on their own behalf or if they have been assigned the task of communication by someone else. This ensures that the receiver of the call has a clear idea as to whether the call has been instigated at an appropriate level; this helps to avoid misunderstandings later on.

## What is needed (from the listener)

This is the most important part of the call from the perspective of both the caller and the listener. It is therefore essential that the need is stated clearly and succinctly. To ensure that this is the case a little time needs to be taken before the call is initiated to clarify the exact requirement in terms of both personnel and services.

## What are the (relevant) patient details

The exact details that are relevant will vary with the nature of the need. However, a minimum data set consists of:

- patient's full name
- patient's date of birth
- current location.

## What the problem is

This is closely related to the need and the details given will vary according to its nature. For example, communications designed to book an intensive care bed will be very different from those to an ambulance service to arrange transportation. In the first example considerable clinical information will be required and the exact amount will be a matter of negotiation between the instigator and receiver of the call. This negotiation is an important aspect of the call; the instigator should prepare a concise verbal presentation of the clinical details and should also ensure that the receiving unit is informed about any other potentially relevant patient details. Any other potentially useful information should be to hand as well. There is nothing more irritating when receiving a telephone referral than to have every request for additional information followed by a pause and a question to a third party shouted in the background.

## What has been done to address the problem and what happened

If the communication is designed to obtain clinical services then the therapy given, and the response to that treatment, will be very important to the receiver of the call who must assure themselves that all appropriate measures have been undertaken. This is especially important when the referral is to a specialist service, since the delivery of good care early will help to ensure that the patient arrives in the best possible condition.

## What is needed (from the listener) – again

Since the statement of need is so important it is recommended that it is restated at the end of the communication so that no misunderstandings occur.

# COMMUNICATION METHODS

The communication methods used during the transfer process are the same as those used during day to day practice. The usual method within the clinical area instigating the transfer is face to face speech, while most other communications (within both the instigating hospital and the receiving unit) are by phone, both land line and cellular. Occasionally it will be necessary to use radios; the practical aspects of this are dealt with in Chapter 9.

# WRITTEN RECORDS

Written records are especially important from both clinical and legal perspectives. Apart from a few taped calls, written notes are usually the only records that remain once the transfer is completed. They must be as accurate as possible and should include as a minimum:

- patient details
- timings
- clinical baseline history and examination
- clinical interventions and effects of these interventions
- investigations carried out and their results
- condition during transfer
- names of responsible clinicians at each stage of the transfer.

Much of this can be achieved by attaching a structured transfer record to the clinical notes. One such record is shown in Figure 4.1.

**Summary**

Clear and effective communication and recording is an essential part of the transfer process.

| ICU TRANSFER FORM<br>INSTRUCTIONS FOR USE OF THIS FORM<br>To be used for all patients transferred to ICU – this is a legal record of transfer | | Time | | | | | | | | | | | | |
|---|---|---|---|---|---|---|---|---|---|---|---|---|---|---|
| **PATIENT DETAILS** | **TRANSFER DETAILS** | Drugs | | | | | | | | | | | | |
| | | Monitoring<br>SaO$_2$<br>ETCO$_2$ | | | | | | | | | | | | |
| Audit data: | | 220<br>200<br>180<br>160<br>140<br>120.... | | | | | | | | | | | | |
| **HISTORY & CLINICAL FINDINGS** | | Fluids | | | | | | | | | | | | |
| | | Please list any precautions taken for fractured spine at any level | | | | | | | | | | | | |
| **STABILISATION TIME** | **AMBULANCE DETAILS** | TRANSFER COMMENTS/PROBLEMS: | | | | | | | | | | | | |
| **STAFF ARRANGING TRANSFER** | **ESCORTING PERSONNEL** | | | | | | | | | | | | | |
| At transferring hospital | Doctor | COMMENTS OF RECEIVING DOCTOR: | | | | | | | | | | | | |
| At recipient hospital | Nurse/ODA | | | | | | | | | | | | | |
| **VENTILATION DURING TRANSFER** | **MONITORING** | Signature of receiving doctor: | | | | | | | | | | | | |

**Figure 4.1.** ICU transfer form.

CHAPTER

# 5

# Evaluation

---

**Objectives**

- Understand how to recognise and agree the need for transfer.
- Understand how to evaluate the transfer category.

---

Evaluation is a dynamic process which starts from first contact with the patient. The aims are to decide whether transfer is appropriate and, if it is, the priority of the patient in comparison with others in your hospital. By the time the assessment, control, and communication have been completed enough information will have been gathered to enable evaluation to be carried out.

## RECOGNISING AND AGREEING THE NEED FOR TRANSFER

The possibility of transfer on clinical grounds should occur to the team at the primary hospital as the diagnosis unfolds. This requires recognition that the needs of the patient may be better met elsewhere. In order to make this decision the likely or possible diagnoses, must be identified and the best treatment for such a condition must be known. The lack of local facilities, resources or personnel to make the definitive diagnosis, and/or to treat the condition optimally must be recognised and suitable acceptable alternatives must be sought.

Referral patterns and common indications for clinical transfers will be well known in most units. In the past the majority of transfers were for conditions which were best managed by regional or supraregional specialists. Increasingly, though, referrals are being made because no ICU bed is currently available within the originating hospital. This is a simple capacity problem. In a minority of cases, patients require transfer to their home area or country.

Having flagged up the possible need for transfer, the clinician at the receiving centre should be contacted. A two-way dialogue will usually result in an agreement that transfer is appropriate. Sometimes immediate agreement is not possible and further information is required. For example, a neurosurgeon may need to assess a CT scan transmitted electronically from the referring centre. Occasionally agreement is not achieved because of hopeless prognosis (for example, 80% burns in an elderly patient) or is deferred until stabilisation has been achieved to permit safe transfer.

After agreeing the appropriateness of transfer, the receiving clinician must check that the receiving centre is physically able to accept the patient. Necessary resources (such as intensive care beds) should be currently available. An exception to this rule is when the nearest receiving centre has the capability to perform a life saving surgical intervention which is critically time dependent. In such a situation, transfer prior to availability of resources may be justified but the specialist receiving centre may have to arrange further transfer postoperatively.

# THE TRANSFER CATEGORY

This is the next stage in the process and part of the dialogue between the referring and the receiving clinicians. The need for extra treatment prior to or during transfer should be discussed and an assessment of the urgency of transfer should be made. A primary goal of safe transfer is to move the appropriate treatment environment with the patient. Thus, for transfer of an intensive care patient, the ambulance should function as a mobile ICU.

A useful tool for determining the appropriate transfer needs is the Transfer Category Table (Figure 5.1). The patient's illness or injury is categorised in such a way as to incorporate severity and urgency. It provides a consistent method of allocating resources (vehicle, escorts, and equipment) and defining the ambulance response time.

The clinical urgency is divided into six categories.

> **Categories of clinical urgency**
>
> - Intensive
> - Time critical
> - Ill and unstable
> - Ill and stable
> - Unwell
> - Well

## Intensive

Though intensive patients are usually the most complicated (often requiring ventilation and invasive monitoring), they are not necessarily the most urgent. Careful stabilisation prior to transfer is important.

In most cases, a time of 20 minutes for the ambulance to be made available is appropriate. It takes almost this long to establish the patient on a transport ventilator and repeat blood gas analysis to confirm appropriate settings. It remains important to order the ambulance proactively to avoid unnecessary delay once the ambulance arrives. An example of such a case is a child with severe meningococcal septicaemia requiring transfer from a level 2 to a level 3 facility. Resuscitation fluids, inotropes, and antibiotics will have been given already. Arterial and central venous lines will have been established and intubation will usually have been performed. Intensive patients will often require advanced respiratory support and advanced monitoring techniques. Frequently more than one organ system will need supporting. The transfer team should include an intensive care doctor and a nurse trained in critical care.

| Degree of illness | Vehicle | Personnel | | | | Extra equipment | Urgency |
|---|---|---|---|---|---|---|---|
| | | Ambulance | Nursing | Medical | Other carer | | |
| Intensive | Single cot emergency ambulance with: • stretcher • siren • speed • suction • oxygen • Basic Life Support kit • defibrillator | Driver-porter or technician | Trained nurse + critical care experience from sending or receiving unit | ICU-trained doctor of at least specialist registrar level | Occasionally intensive care technician or operating department practitioner | • Advanced Life Support kit • ventilator • monitor • syringe pump • extra drugs | 20 minutes but <10 if immediate intervention required in receiving area |
| Time critical | | Advanced Life Support practitioner (paramedic or enhanced nurse) with driver-porter or technician. Nurse from sending unit if no other nurse in team | | According to perceived risk | If necessary for safety or to prevent distress, primary carer from own home, nursing home or institution | • Advanced Life Support kit • monitor • syringe pump | 8 minutes |
| Ill and unstable | | | | | | | 30 minutes |
| Ill and stable | | Basic Life Support practitioner (technician or trained nurse) with driver-porter. Nurse from sending unit if no other nurse in team | | | | • often monitor • occasional syringe pump | 60 minutes |
| Unwell | Patient transport (PTS) vehicle | First-Aider and other attendant including driver | | | | • first aid kit • oxygen • pocket mask | 120 minutes |
| Well | PTS vehicle or taxi or car | Driver | | | | | As available |

**Figure 5.1.** Transfer category table.

## Time critical

Time critical transfers involve patients requiring the most urgent transportation. These transfers require a similar response time from the ambulance service as a 999 call. An example is a patient with evidence of a ruptured abdominal aortic aneurysm with no facilities to perform surgery on site. Delaying to attempt stabilisation is of little or no benefit. Transferring such patients requires an advanced life support provider, who may be a paramedic, an enhanced trained nurse or a doctor. Not all critical transfers will require a doctor.

## Ill and unstable

These patients require urgent transfer but a response time of up to 30 minutes is generally acceptable.

An ill and unstable patient requires an advanced life support provider as an escort. A doctor may be required, depending on the perceived risk and the expected duration of the journey.

Critical and ill and unstable patients will often need additional respiratory support (such as oxygen or an oropharyngeal airway) and additional monitoring (such as a continuous ECG trace, pulse oximetry, and blood pressure measurement).

A patient with acute gastrointestinal bleeding, which is settling but which has a high risk of recurrence, is in this category. Other examples include patients with an acutely perforated duodenal ulcer, repeated seizures vulnerable to relapse or unstable cardiac arrhythmias.

## Ill and stable

Transfer within 60 minutes is desirable.

Ill and stable patients constitute the majority of medical and surgical patients admitted to hospital for acute care on a daily basis. Examples include patients with a chest infection without serious respiratory compromise, a stroke without airway obstruction, irregular breathing or hypotension or acute appendicitis without perforation.

They are considered stable enough not to require the presence of an advanced life support provider en route if transferred. Nevertheless, basic life support skills will be needed. These patients are ill and will require a stretcher rather than a seat in an ambulance. Most hospitals consider that all ill patients require an accompanying nurse for any transfer.

## Unwell and well

Patients classified as unwell or well are included in the table for completeness but will not be discussed further here. They form an important part of the overall transport requirement within a large hospital (especially intrahospital rather than interhospital transfer) but require no special arrangements.

**Summary**

The need for transfer and the category of transfer must be agreed.

# 6

# Preparation and packaging

**Objectives**

- Understand the preparation of the patient, the equipment, and the personnel.
- Understand the packaging of the patient.

## INTRODUCTION

Whilst it is not possible to provide all aspects of critical care support during a transfer, this does not mean that the standards of monitoring and management should be deliberately reduced. In fact, with adequate preparation most advanced care can continue throughout. To achieve this, both the current needs of the patient and their potential needs en route, should be considered. Before leaving, the patient must be packaged, by fully protecting and securing all equipment and implementing measures to reduce the effects of the hostile environment.

## PREPARATION

There are three distinct areas that require preparation before packaging can be commenced. First, the patient must be stabilised to reduce physiological complications during the journey; second, all the necessary equipment must be found and checked; and finally, the personnel who are to undertake the transfer must be fully prepared.

### Patient preparation

Prior to the transfer taking place the team leader must ensure that the patient is in the best possible condition and that all team members are fully briefed about his/her needs.

The patient must have a "definitive" airway. If there is any doubt whatsoever about the patient's airway or conscious level, then elective intubation should be undertaken prior to departure. As a guide, anyone with a GCS < 9 should be intubated prior to transfer, unless there is a good reason not to do so. The need to intubate en route should arise very rarely.

The cervical spine should be immobilised in patients with either inadequately assessed or known unstable neck injury. Hard collar and blocks should be used. In those patients without cervical injury, it is still often necessary to stabilise the head prior to a rapid transfer. While simple measures such as bags of fluid placed either side of the head stop the head rolling, they offer little real cervical spine protection.

Spontaneously breathing patients will require a non-rebreathing mask with high flow oxygen. These types of patient are usually much better sat up.

Chest drains can present a major problem. Underwater seal bottles are cumbersome, they can tip over and spill, and must never be clamped. If drainage is minimal, then good alternatives are simple one-way valve drainage bags.

At least two reliable sites of intravenous access should be available. One should be the route for fluid volume replacement. This line should have a "blood giving" set attached and a full bag of fluid put up just prior to departure. The line needs to be threaded out of the "mummy wrap" (see below) for easy access. The second line can be flushed and turned off. This line can be left inside the wrap.

For shorter transfers (< 20 minutes), maintenance fluids may sometimes be ignored. However, if required, an infusion pump or syringe driver will be far more effective than a drip set, whilst in motion. Infusion pumps are large, heavy, and far from ideal for transfers. Syringe drivers are a less cumbersome alternative but less suited for large volume infusions unfortunately though, infusions may therefore need to be delivered in a more concentrated solution via syringes for the journey.

Sedation and inotropes should be rationalised so as to take the least possible number of infusions. Some sedation can be given by bolus injection and even ICU patients rarely require more than three infusions.

Any suspicion of a spinal injury, at any level, warrants spinal immobilisation during transport. This makes patient handling much easier but stability on top of the ambulance stretcher must be checked prior to departure. There is a high incidence of pressure sores with prolonged spinal board use. Vacuum mattresses offer a useful alternative. All fractures must be immobilised prior to transport. Be aware that some fixators and traction devices may not fit into the transport vehicle and they may require modification or removal.

A detailed observation chart should be started as early as possible. Maintaining the chart can be assigned to the escorting nurse if necessary.

Patients frequently become relatively hypothermic whilst being stabilised for transfer. The use of warm air, quilts, and efforts to minimise the time spent exposed during invasive procedures will reduce heat losses.


## Equipment preparation

*Patient equipment*

The transport equipment should not be used for anything else. It should be stored in a specific location and must be checked regularly. Monitors and pumps must be kept fully charged. Some items may be stored separately, for example, drugs that are stored cold, warmed fluids, controlled drugs, and batteries on charge; these can easily be forgotten. It is therefore important to check everything. A loading list or series of photographs may help.

Many units use transport rucksacks that can be unzipped all the way round and laid out flat. These can hold large amounts of equipment and are very portable. In the confines of an ambulance or aircraft rucksacks with single compartments can be very awkward to open and access. In these instances multi-compartment bags have proven very successful. A number of these bags also contain smaller pouch-bags with specific roles such as "airway" or "intravenous access". When moving critically ill patients over long distances, a great deal of equipment may be required. To spread the load, two smaller transport packs are often better than one large one.

After each transfer, the medical and nursing staff must go through the equipment and replace any items used. During a transfer, it may help to keep a record of any items used.

The kit must contain all means of manually supporting the airway and full intubation equipment. This should include a selection of sizes of airways, endotracheal tubes, and an emergency cricothyroidotomy set. Effective portable suction must be available at all times. Hand or foot operated units can be very efficient for large volume suction and have the advantage of needing no external power or gas supply.

The kit should contain everything necessary to deliver oxygen to a self-ventilating patient. Oxygen supply can be one of the greatest problems during longer transports. A simple oxygen consumption calculation should be made prior to departure. This must be based upon the likely travel time and the flow rate or minute volume of the patient.

$$\text{Minute volume} = \text{tidal volume} \times \text{respiratory rate}$$

The flow rates necessary to obtain various $FIO_2$ targets through a ventimask are shown in Table 6.1. The gas consumption of a self-inflating bag system is difficult to predict. A Waters (Mapleton C) circuit requires a gas flow three times the minute volume to prevent rebreathing.

**Table 6.1.** Flow rates for ventimasks

|  | % Oxygen | | | | |
| --- | --- | --- | --- | --- | --- |
|  | 24 | 28 | 35 | 40 | 60 |
| Flow rate (l/min) | 2 | 4 | 8 | 10 | 15 |

Ideally for patients requiring ventilatory support a mechanical ventilator should be used. This must be durable, safe, and reliable. Most of the suitable portable ventilators are oxygen driven, providing either 100% oxygen or an air mix that usually has an $FIO_2$ of 45% or so. Most ventilators will use 1 litre/minute "driving gas".

Small transport ventilators such as Transpac™, Ventipac™, Pneupac™, and Oxylog™ use differing volumes of oxygen depending on whether they are set for air mix or no air mix. No air mix consumes the patient's minute volume of oxygen while air mix consumes one third of the patient's minute volume.

Intensive care patients require a ventilator that can cope with a variety of pulmonary states. PEEP facilities should be considered a minimum.

The estimated oxygen requirements can be calculated by multiplying the predicted journey time in minutes by the minute volume. The number of cylinders required can simply be calculated by dividing estimated consumption by cylinder capacity. A reserve supply is essential to cover any misadventure en route. Double the estimated consumption is probably the safest option.

**Table 6.2.** Oxygen cylinder capacity.

|  | | Size | |
| --- | --- | --- | --- |
|  | D | E | F |
| Volume (l) | 340 | 680 | 1360 |

The capacity of the three common oxygen cylinders is shown in Table 6.2.

For long road transfers, the ambulance may have to stop en route at a hospital or ambulance station to collect more oxygen. The reserve can be seen to be especially important when transporting from isolated locations, where additional supplies cannot be collected during the journey.

Specialised transfers may require further equipment checks, e.g. incubators, ECMO machines, portable balloon pumps. These are very specialised areas that may necessitate a skilled technician joining the team. The additional team member must be fully briefed on the patient, the transfer, and details of the mode of transport, e.g. power and gas supplies on board.

*Staff equipment*

All the transport team must be adequately equipped to cope with the weather otherwise they will be uncomfortable and perform badly. Protective clothing should be appropriate to the situation. As well as warmth and visibility, head, eye, and ear protection may also be necessary.

Individual members of the team require personal equipment. A simple mnemonic checklist is shown in Box 6.1.

---

**Box 6.1.   Personal equipment**

| | |
| --- | --- |
| P | Phone |
| E | Enquiry number and name |
| R | Revenue |
| S | Safe clothing |
| O | Organised route |
| N | Nutrition |
| A | A–Z |
| L | Lift home |

---

The telephone allows direct communication with both the receiving and home unit.

A map is essential as it is not unknown for vehicles to get lost, particularly when they are travelling outside the region. In the event of a long journey, food and refreshment should be carried together with the resources to either get home or stay overnight in safe accommodation.

## Personnel preparation

As a basic minimum, staff involved in transferring must have current advanced life support skills and should have skills in critical care. They need to be familiar with the patient's condition and the drugs currently in progress. They must also be familiar with the selected mode of transport and know why they are going.

Good communication between transport staff is essential in order to allocate responsibilities and prevent duplication.

# PACKAGING

Any endotracheal tube must be securely fastened. This usually means a cord tie or cotton tape (see Chapter 8) but care must be taken to avoid neck compression, especially in head injured patients. Children have relatively hypermobile mandibles and therefore tubes should not be fastened to the jaw. The maxillae offer a much more reliable point of attachment. Ideally, all small children should have a nasal rather than an oral tube, as this can be made very secure, with Elastoplast "trousers". However, nasal intubation is a very skilled procedure and should never be attempted by the inexperienced, especially in an unwell child. Anaesthetists with paediatric critical care training will pass an oral tube and then replace it with a nasal. In skilled hands the benefits of this technique usually outweigh the risks.

All endotracheal tubes should be cut to the correct length, as excessively long tubes will tend to kink, especially when attached to a ventilator circuit. Small sized paediatric tubes are at much greater risk of this and may need tape around the tube to add some rigidity.

At all stages when the patient is being transferred, the endotracheal tube must be monitored so as to prevent extubation. This is a particular risk when moving from bed to stretcher. If the patient will tolerate a short period of disconnection, then this is the safest way to avoid inadvertent extubation during such manoeuvres.

If the atmospheric pressure is likely to change significantly, for example during air transport, the cuff on the tube may be better filled with saline rather than air, which avoids the associated volume changes which can damage the trachea.

It is useful to protect the eyes of sedated patients, with tape or gauze. This should prevent accidental corneal abrasion but must still allow visualisation of the pupils, to assess sedation levels.

Ventilators and associated equipment need very careful checking prior to departure. All the transport team must be familiar with the particular ventilator in use and all its alarms. The ventilator should be mounted above the patient on a platform or fastened securely to the side of the stretcher. It must be clearly visible and easy to reach at all times. The contents gauge of the oxygen supply must also be clearly visible and monitored regularly. A reserve oxygen supply must be readily to hand and should have an appropriate connector attached. In addition, a cylinder key is considered an essential part of the kit and needs to be readily available. Ventilators and cylinders must be securely fastened for transport.

Adequacy of respiratory support is assessed by pulse oximetry and capnography (see Chapter 8). The oximeter probe can be placed on a finger inside the "mummy wrap", as in this low light it is more likely to work well. Taping the probe to the finger can lead to pressure necrosis. Self-adhesive probes are very useful and function well in vibrating environments. Ear probes are rarely of value for transport purposes. Capnography is especially important to maintain a low–normal $pCO_2$ in cases of potentially raised intracranial pressure. Ventilator pressure and disconnect alarms are notoriously difficult to hear during transport. If fitted, they should be used but they do not offer an alternative to being extra vigilant in transit.

When the patient is wrapped prior to transfer, one point of venous access should be kept easily available to avoid delays giving drugs. Jugular and subclavian central lines often provide good points of access for a carer sitting at the head of the patient. The access port can be secured to the pillow or shoulder of the patient to avoid displacement during the journey.

Many monitors are required to assess the patient's physiological status. This results in a potentially huge jumble of cables and wires. To avoid this all the leads should be brought together as one bundle. This can be protected with some split plastic tubing or tubular bandage. The whole bundle can be threaded out of the "mummy wrap", at either the head or the feet, to the monitor.

Invasive pressure lines must be flushed and zeroed prior to use. They are accurate, less sensitive to vibration and rapidly detect changes in pressure. However, they must be kept bubble free and heparinised. Sets are now available which do not require cumbersome pressure bags. Pressure transducers can be fastened, one to each upper arm. Here they are readily accessible for flushing and zeroing. They are also at an appropriate level for monitoring cardiac pressures. Gauze should be placed under each transducer before taping to the arm, to prevent pressure necrosis. After securing the transducers, all the connections in the pressure set should be retightened to avoid disconnection en route.

The power for monitors and pumps can often be drawn from the ambulance or aircraft. This requires prior discussion with the transport vehicle operator, particularly for air transport since special arrangements may be required.

Heat loss outside the warm hospital environment presents a major problem. This can be substantially reduced by "mummy wrapping" the patient (see Chapter 8). Patients can be wrapped in prewarmed blankets and then covered with an insulating layer. Alternatively, special quilts or sleeping bags can be used for maximal insulation. These also ensure that, once wrapped, the patient is very neatly packaged, avoiding lots of loose leads and lines.

The environment inside the transport vehicle should also be considered. It may be possible to heat or cool the patient area or to reduce noise or movement in some way.

Stretchers should ideally have a number of securing straps for the patient and provision for head blocks. A platform device for bulky equipment such as monitors and ventilators should be available. Ideally, this needs to sit across the patient during transport but be able to be lifted off when required. This avoids the need to lay equipment upon the patient's legs.

**Summary**

Adequate preparation of the patient, the equipment, and the transport personnel, together with attention to the details of packaging, will ensure that the transportation phase itself has the best chance of being free of adverse events.

# 7

# Transportation

## INTRODUCTION

Transportation takes place in three distinct phases. First, the patient is moved from the referring unit to the transferring vehicle. Second, the vehicle, team, and patient move from the referring to the receiving unit. Finally, the patient is moved from the transferring vehicle to the receiving unit trolley or bed. These three phases are dealt with separately below.

## LEAVING THE REFERRING UNIT

The patient and transfer team should be fully prepared and packaging must be complete before any movement is initiated. A final check should be carried out to ensure that no final actions are required to ensure optimum resuscitation. In addition, a final check should be made to ensure that tubes, drains, and lines are as secure as possible. Box 7.1 shows the sequence of actions that should occur.

**Box 7.1. Checklist prior to leaving the referring unit**

- Move the transport trolley next to the bed and match heights.
- Uncover the patient.
    - If breathing spontaneously, change to transport oxygen supply and ensure mask is appropriate and fitting.

– If requiring ventilation, ensure the transport oxygen cylinder has the appropriate valve.

– Or hand ventilate using 100% oxygen.

- Ensure adequate ventilation both sides of the chest.
- Ensure any chest drain is secure and functioning.
- Check that any bandages providing tamponade are secure.
- Ensure lines are secure, untangled, and functioning.
- Hang up any fluid bags so they will not interfere with the transfer of the patient.
- Ensure upper limbs are kept adducted by assistant or Velcro strapping.
- Check the position of the urinary catheter and position it between the patient's legs.
- Check the position of the naso/orogastric tube and position the bag on the patient's chest.
- Warn patient.
- Check that no line or tube is likely to be snared in the move.
- Move the patient to the transport trolley using appropriate aids.

# MOVEMENT BETWEEN UNITS

The aim is to provide seamless, appropriate care throughout. To achieve this a series of pretransfer checks should be carried out and problems should be dealt with swiftly if they arise.

## Airway

Loss of control of the airway in any patient may result in a serious hypoxic event. Failure to recognise that a problem has developed can therefore have fatal consequences. During transportation, space constraints and subsequent lack of access can result in difficult airway assessment. It is essential that a member of the transfer team is capable of recognising airway threats and is competent to deal with any problems that arise.

---

**Box 7.2.  Pretransfer checklist: airway**

- Is it possible to assess the airway?
- Is there a member of the team present who can secure that airway, if required?

If the patient is intubated

- Is the endotracheal tube visible?
- Is the pilot balloon visible?
- Are the connections to the ventilation tubing visible?
- Does a member of the team have access to any drugs and equipment that might be needed?

---

*Endotracheal tube dislodgement*

The endotracheal tube may become dislodged or slip further in, particularly if it is not secured adequately. To prevent this, not only should the endotracheal tube be secured to the patient but the ventilator circuit must also be safe from traction or tension.

The usual disconnect monitors may not be available and normal visualisation of the patient may not be possible. Furthermore, most standard transportation ventilators do not have a means to measure expired volumes from a patient's lungs.

> **Action**
>
> - Stop the moving vehicle if possible and assess the patient.
> - Confirm displacement by direct visualisation.
> - Ventilate via bag-valve-mask technique.
> - With all the appropriate equipment available, reintubate and secure endotracheal tube.

### Tracheal cuff leak

If the inflated cuff of an endotracheal tube starts to leak patient safety can be compromised. Significant loss of inspired minute ventilation from a ventilator will result in hypoventilation and eventual hypoxia and hypercarbia. A leak around a deflated cuff allows secretions, blood, and gastric contents to contaminate the bronchial tree.

> **Action**
>
> - Attempt to introduce more air/saline into the cuff.
> - If the pilot balloon is damaged, introduce more air/saline into the cuff and clamp the pilot tube with artery forceps.
> - If the pilot balloon is lost consider introducing a 22G cannula into the pilot tube and reinflating the balloon.
> - Replace the endotracheal tube completely.

### Tracheal tube obstruction

This can occur as a result of secretions drying within the endotracheal tube, often through the use of dry oxygen to ventilate the patient's lungs. An increase in inflation pressure may be seen on the ventilator when there is an obstruction within the tube. Failure to overcome this obstruction can result in inadequate ventilation of the patient's lungs, especially when dealing with the small diameter tubes needed for paediatric patients. Use of a humidifier and moisture exchanger may reduce this complication.

> **Action**
>
> - Use the suction device and an appropriate suction catheter to clear secretions from the endotracheal tube lumen.
> - Replace the endotracheal tube completely.

### Drugs

To ensure an endotracheal tube can be tolerated, the patient must be adequately sedated (and paralysed when necessary).

> **Action**
>
> - Ensure sufficient amounts of sedation are available for the transfer.
> - Ensure a reliable intravenous site for delivery.
> - Ensure battery lives of infusion pumps are adequate for the journey.

## Breathing

A patient covered in blankets and strapped to a trolley or stretcher will not be easy to assess for symmetrical chest movements. Any inadvertent movement of the endotracheal tube can easily result in endobronchial intubation and subsequent hypoxia. This is particularly a problem with small, uncuffed tubes in paediatric transfers.

---

**Box 7.3.  Pretransfer checklist: breathing**

If the patient is ventilated:

- can you see symmetrical chest movement?
- can you assess how adequately the patient is ventilated?
- do you have access to the patient?
- do you have direct visual access to the ventilator and monitors?

---

Measuring arterial $CO_2$ is not practical during the transfer. Measuring end-tidal $CO_2$ using capnography, however, will give a constant indication of the adequacy of ventilation. The capnograph can also act as an extremely sensitive disconnection alarm since the trace will disappear once the patient is no longer ventilated. This is important since the normal alarm system of the ventilator is unlikely to be effective during transport. At altitude, changes in barometric pressure affect the $CO_2$ readings from the capnograph. Some monitors have an inbuilt altimeter to compensate for atmospheric pressure changes.

Lung ventilation and perfusion mismatch can occur during transfer since the blood flow in the relatively low pressure system of the lung is influenced by centripetal and acceleration/deceleration forces. This may result in the patient becoming hypoxic. Extra oxygen must be added to compensate for the increasing intrapulmonary shunting of deoxygenated blood. Thus, for all but the most stable adult patients, it is wise to increase the inspired oxygen concentration during the transfer.

Pulse oximetry gives a continuous measurement of the level of tissue oxygenation at the probe site. It is a reliable monitor but may be adversely affected during transfer. If the patient is cold and peripherally vasoconstricted, the signal strength may not be sufficient to give an accurate reading of oxygen saturation. Furthermore, readings can be distorted by vibration artefact and excessive ambient light.

*Loss of oxygen supply*

Loss of oxygen supply not only reduces the $FIO_2$ but also stops the ventilator working altogether since most transport ventilators are gas powered. Prevention is much better than cure and although some causes, such as faulty seals, are unpredictable, the commonest cause (failure to take enough oxygen) is.

---

**Action**

- Calculate the amount of oxygen required before departing.
- Know where the cylinder key is stored.
- Keep spare seals in your transfer equipment.
- Have a self-inflating bag available at all times.

---

*Pneumothorax*

Pneumothorax can be life threatening in a ventilated patient but is difficult to confirm in a moving ambulance or aircraft. Noise levels make any attempt to assess air entry into the lung by auscultation with a stethoscope futile. A rise in the inflation pressure on the ventilator dial may be the only sign that a pneumothorax has developed. Unless steps are taken at this stage, a tension pneumothorax may ensue. A pre-existing chest drain can give a false sense of security since a pleural leak can occur at another site or the existing chest drain can obstruct.

---

**Action**

- React early to any rise in inflation pressure.
- Avoid glass bottles and underwater sealed drains.
- Stop and check the patient if suspicion arises.

---

*Capnography*

Mainstream capnographs can be affected by moisture build-up within the sampling window and this can lead to distortion of the recorded trace.

---

**Action**

- Attach sampling system with detection "window" upright to avoid condensed moisture collecting within it.

---

## Circulation

The near constant presence of changing forces of acceleration and deceleration, as well as centripetal effects, can result in rapid venous pooling of blood in the peripheral tissues. This results in apparent relative hypovolaemia. Again, prevention is better than cure and it is important to ensure that the patient is at least normovolaemic prior to commencing transfer.

---

**Box 7.4. Pretransfer checklist: circulation**

- Can you assess the patient's circulatory situation?
- Do you have adequate IV access?
- Can you respond to change in the patient's circulatory status?

---

Non-invasive blood pressure cuff readings are not able to give a "real time" view of changes in blood pressure. The cuff pressure readings can be distorted by excessive vibration and non-invasive cuff readings result in a greater drain on the power source. It is more effective to monitor cardiovascular parameters by using invasive pressure lines. Direct arterial and central venous pressure monitoring gives the transfer team immediate information. Transducers should be secured to the patient at an appropriate level (see Chapter 6) since access may be impossible during the transfer.

The urinary catheter bag should be emptied (and the volume recorded) prior to transfer so that it does not compromise the limited space on the transport trolley.

Depending on the length of the transfer, the hourly urine output should be monitored throughout the transfer.

Any crossmatched blood should be transferred in an appropriate cool box, along with the laboratory crossmatch forms. It may be of benefit to check with the receiving unit that they are willing to accept the blood from you, rather than potentially wasting a valuable resource.

*Loss of invasive monitor waveforms*

Any invasive line can obstruct with thrombus if not flushed effectively. If a pressure waveform disappears from the screen, the patient should be checked for clinical deterioration immediately.

> **Action**
>
> - Check pressure bags are inflated to an appropriate level and all the connections along the flush line are secure to the transducer.
> - Check that the transducer will register a pressure rise when the line is flushed manually.
> - Ensure the cable interface to your monitor is connected.

*Monitor or pump power failure*

All monitors and pumps can potentially suffer power failure in transit. NiCad replacement batteries can be carried but they are heavy and require extra space. Older NiCad batteries often fail to hold charge to the full extent of the quoted duration.

> **Action**
>
> - Have replacement batteries available and be aware of how to replace them.
> - Carry an inverter on transfers. This allows use of DC power from a vehicle/aircraft battery.
> - Increase the concentration of the inotrope to prolong the syringe lifespan or carry premixed syringes of inotropes to allow easy exchange.

## Disability

An unconscious patient needs regular neurological assessment. However, in a moving ambulance or aircraft this will be very limited.

> **Box 7.5.  Pretransfer checklist: disability**
>
> - Can you assess the patient's neurological status?
> - Can you respond to changes in the patient's neurological status?

A member of the transfer team should be positioned so as to be able to inspect pupillary responses to light. A handheld light source should be available for this.

The position of the eyes and response of the pupils may be the only clinical sign available to confirm elevated intracranial pressure. In addition, the only evidence of an underlying convulsion in the paralysed patient may be abnormally responding pupils.

Ideally, the level of paralysis should be monitored with a nerve stimulator. However, access to limbs may be limited and facial twitches can be difficult to interpret during transit.

Rapid changes in acceleration and deceleration forces will result in rises in intracranial pressure that can compromise cerebral perfusion. Maintaining a constant speed and minimising sudden turns is therefore beneficial when transferring a patient with a traumatic brain injury. Even if the patient's cervical spine has been cleared radiologically, it may be useful to secure the patient's head to avoid twisting or turning, which can impair venous drainage from an already compromised brain.

## Exposure and environment

---

**Box 7.6.   Pretransfer checklist: exposure and environment**

- Is the patient adequately covered and secured?
- Is the monitoring and therapeutic equipment adequately secured?
- Are all personnel adequately secured?

---

The transporting vehicle can be a hostile place for both patient and transfer personnel. Low ambient temperature may render the unconscious patient hypothermic since a thermo-neutral environment is often difficult to achieve. Their temperature can fall further during the often protracted process of moving to and from vehicles.

There is a constant risk from unsecured equipment during transfer. It is therefore important that all non-essential equipment is stored away, when not in use. Any heavy monitoring equipment should be strapped securely to surrounding framework.

All personnel should be restrained securely whilst moving. The transfer team are at risk from nausea and vomiting, which can easily impair their vigilance during a transfer. An associated phenomenon, known as Sopite syndrome, results in the transfer personnel having a desire to withdraw from the environment as well as suffering from abdominal discomfort. Those suffering with the collection of symptoms that are associated with this syndrome have been shown to have reduced psychometric testing scores.

## Monitoring

Capnography, pulse oximetry, and invasive pressure monitoring have been considered earlier in this chapter and are dealt with in detail in Chapter 8. In addition to these, many other forms of monitoring may be appropriate during transfer.

The ECG should be monitored routinely during critical care transfer. At least three electrodes are required, allowing two for sensing and a ground. Some monitors use more electrodes to allow flexible switching between leads. The electrodes should be placed appropriately to facilitate interpretation. Positioning them to provide the equivalent of standard leads II and V5 is useful for detecting P-waves/arrhythmias and myocardial ischaemia respectively.

Non-invasive blood pressure and temperature monitoring (e.g. nasopharyngeal, oesophageal or rectal) should be considered during transfer. Both parameters are easily measured and are available on many portable monitors. The former is generally regarded as inferior to invasive arterial pressure for transferring critically ill or injured patients but it is still wise to take a cuff as a back-up technique.

Central venous pressure is measured using the same technology as invasive arterial pressure. If the transport monitor has two invasive pressure channels, both may be displayed en route. If only one is available, arterial monitoring is generally more valuable. Even in this situation, the central venous pressure may be measured intermittently by switching momentarily from the arterial trace, using a male to male connector to connect the three-way taps on the arterial and venous tubing.

Most portable ventilators show airway pressure on a mechanical dial or digital display. Not all such ventilators have pressure alarms, though these should now be regarded as mandatory. They need to indicate when the pressure is too low, suggesting an airway disconnection or leak. They should also indicate when it is too high, so as to warn of tension pneumothorax or airway obstruction (from tube kinking, bronchospasm or secretions).

If intracranial pressure (ICP) is being monitored beforehand, this may be continued during transfer. Intraparenchymal fibre optic devices, inserted directly into superficial brain tissue through a very small hole drilled in the skull, are commonly used to measure ICP and generally have an adequate battery for transfer. Be aware that many neurosurgical centres use different devices, so that compatibility of equipment after transfer may be an issue affecting whether or not to insert such a monitor immediately prior to transfer. Checking pupil responses, while clearly less discriminating than ICP, should still be regarded as part of the neurological monitoring during transfer.

Urine output measurements should be continued during transfer, using graduated containers for accurate recording. Particular attention should be paid to emptying the urine container prior to transferring the patient between different trolley/bed surfaces. Otherwise someone may lay the container flat for the transfer across, losing the current aliquot of urine collected. The collecting bag beneath the graduated container should be emptied when it is full, as several litres of fluid within the bag constitute a hazard when manoeuvring.

## ARRIVING AT THE RECEIVING UNIT

A rapid assessment of the patient is required to determine if any immediate action is necessary. In addition, care needs to be taken to ensure that tubes, drains, and lines are not dislodged during the transfer from the trolley to the ICU bed. It is advisable to have a designated team leader so that activities are coordinated and none are forgotten.

Box 7.7 shows the sequence of actions that should occur.

---

**Box 7.7.   Checklist on arrival at the receiving unit**

- Move the trolley next to the bed and match heights.
- Uncover the patient.
  - If breathing spontaneously, change to wall mounted oxygen and ensure mask is appropriate and fitting.
  - If requiring ventilation, ensure the receiving unit is set up appropriately. Either change to the receiving unit ventilator and assess or
  - Hand ventilate using 100% oxygen.
- Ensure adequate ventilation both sides of the chest.
- Ensure any chest drain is secure and functioning.
- Check that any bandages providing tamponade are secure.
- Ensure lines are secure, untangled, and functioning.
- Change any empty fluid bags and hang them up so they will not interfere with the transfer of the patient.
- Ensure upper limbs are kept adducted by assistant or Velcro strapping.
- Check the position of the urinary catheter, empty the bag if full, and position it between the patient's legs.

---

- Check the position of the naso/orogastric tube, empty the bag if full, and position the bag on the patient's chest.
- Warn patient.
- Check that no line or tube is likely to be snared in the move.
- Move the patient to the bed using appropriate aids.
- Reassess the patient in an ABC fashion
  - Recheck the position and function of all tubes, drains and lines.
  - Recheck all monitors.
- In the ventilated patient, take an arterial sample for ABG analysis. Other investigations are dependent upon the patient's condition and the management plan.

**Summary**

Attention to detail at all three stages of the transfer will ensure that the patient is delivered in the best possible condition.

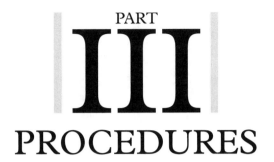

# PART III
# PROCEDURES

CHAPTER

# 8

# Transfer procedures

<br>

**Objectives**

- Describe techniques used to secure equipment.
- Describe appropriate use of monitors.
- Describe the mummy wrap.

## SECURING EQUIPMENT

### IV lines

As a general rule, all venous lines inserted into a patient must be adequately fixed in place prior to transfer. Access lines can be easily dislodged during movement into and out of a vehicle or within the confined space of an ambulance if not well secured and protected.

Peripheral IV cannulae should be fixed in place with either commercially available adhesive dressings or adhesive tape applied to dry skin. A small bandage placed around but not occluding the injection port of the cannula can be useful to help protect it from accidental dislodgement. If an infusion fails, however, the bandage must be removed to ensure that the cannula has not become dislodged. Infusions connected to the cannula can be secured by taping a loop of tubing to the patient, which helps to prevent accidental removal of the cannula.

Central venous lines should *always* be stitched in place after insertion and the insertion sites covered with a transparent, adhesive dressing. Adequate lengths of infusion tubing are needed in order to prevent excessive pulling forces on the cannula.

> Any access line can be accidentally removed during transport if insufficient care is taken to ensure that excessive strains are not placed on the lines and connections.

## Chest drains and endotracheal tubes

*Introduction*

Endotracheal tubes and chest drains obviously play a vital role in the management of patients when used appropriately. Their effectiveness is, however, dependent upon them remaining in position. During transfer they are at risk of becoming dislodged unless they are secured adequately.

Knots play a vital role in ensuring that vital equipment does not become displaced as the patient is transferred.

*Objective*

The aim of tying a knot is to ensure that it is placed where it is required. To do this, tension must not be released until the knot is locked. An example for ET tubes is given below.

*Procedure*
*   Select ribbon gauze for immobilising the endotracheal tube.
*   Each hand should then hold the appropriate end of the tape.
*   Position the tube so that it lies halfway along the length of the tape (see Figure 8.1).

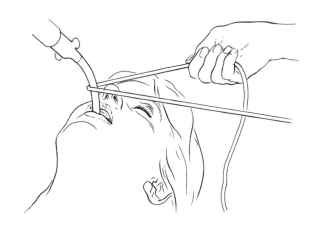

**Figure 8.1.**

*   Keeping the right hand straight, pass the left hand tape over the right hand tape and then up and through the gap; grasp with the left hand (see Figure 8.2).
*   Repeat the procedure (see Figure 8.3).
*   Slide this knot (a slipknot) down the right hand tape and on to the tube at the chosen point (see Figures 8.4 and 8.5).
*   Tighten the knot by pushing the knot with the forefinger of the right hand, whilst pulling the loose ends of the tape (see Figures 8.4 and 8.5).
*   A further slipknot may be fashioned to prevent the knots slipping (see Figures 8.6 and 8.7).

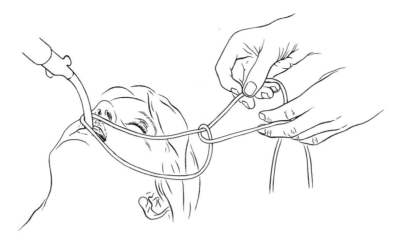

**Figure 8.2.**

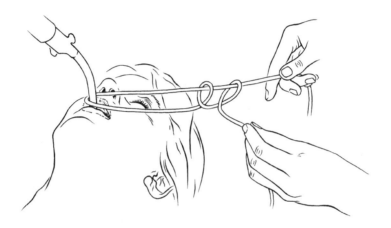

**Figure 8.3.**

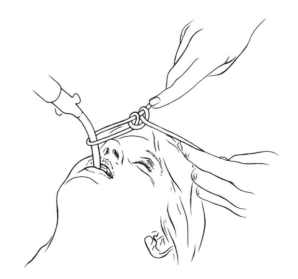

**Figure 8.4.**

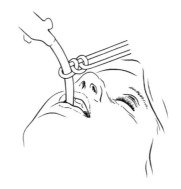

**Figure 8.5.**

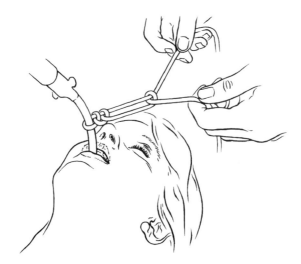

**Figure 8.6.**

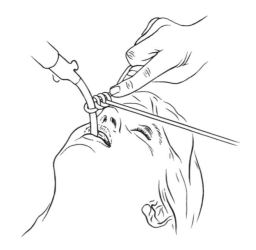

**Figure 8.7.**

- Alternatively use a reverse knot to lock.

---

**Remember**: left over right through and up and reverse to lock securely.

---

- Pass the tape around the back of the neck and secure at the corner of the jaw (see Figure 8.8).

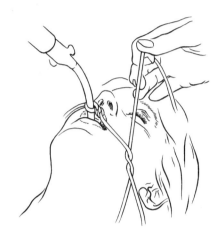

**Figure 8.8.**

## MONITORING

### Pulse oximetry

*Background theory*

Pulse oximetry uses light absorption as a means of estimating arterial oxygen saturation. It is based on the fact that oxyhaemoglobin and deoxyhaemoglobin absorb visible red and invisible infrared electromagnetic radiation differently. The oximeter sends a light signal through a vascular bed, such as a finger or an ear lobe, measures what is transmitted (or reflected) and then uses a computer algorithm to estimate the arterial oxygen saturation. As it is a computer prediction rather than a direct measurement, it is denoted as $SpO_2$ rather than $SaO_2$.

*Set up procedure*

- Switch on the monitor and wait for it to complete the self-test.
- Select a probe which is compatible with the monitor, appropriate for the body part on which it is to be placed and suitable for the age and size of the patient.
- Check that the probe is not damaged and secure it on the patient (finger, ear lobe or other body part, depending on the probe design).
- Ensure that there is a good quality waveform before accepting the value of the $SpO_2$ registered as accurate. If the machine does not have a waveform display, check the intensity scale as an alternative, but much less reliable, quality control signal. Check that the heart rate registered on the pulse oximeter is the same as that on the ECG.

*Clinical problems*

- Vasoconstriction and hypothermia make it difficult to detect a reliable signal from a finger probe. Try alternative probe sites. Check the waveform or intensity scale. The monitor will normally report that the signal is of low strength. Do not rely on the readings in these circumstances.
- Movement and vibration artefact can also result in unreliable readings. As such movement is inevitable during transportation, choose an oximeter with effective noise rejection algorithms.
- If the signal strength is low or the waveform is irregular, check that the probe is properly attached to the patient. If the problem cannot be attributed to poor peripheral perfusion or movement artefact, then check that the probe gives a good signal, a regular waveform, and a normal reading when you place the probe on yourself.
- While a high $SpO_2$ indicates that the blood is well oxygenated, it does not mean that the ventilation is adequate. A low $SpO_2$ may reflect a problem with the patient or with the monitor (measurement artefact). It is wise to assume that the problem is with the patient but still important to check the waveform. In addition, the pulse rate from the pulse oximeter should agree with that from the ECG. If not, this points to an inadequate signal or machine error.
- Irregular pulse rates, especially atrial fibrillation, can impair the oximeter's ability to follow the phases of the pulse cycle, leading to indeterminate or inaccurate readings.
- $SpO_2$ readings are unreliable in the presence of high levels of carboxyhaemoglobin, which absorbs red light in a similar way as oxyhaemoglobin. Take particular care in patients with inhalation injury and carbon monoxide poisoning. High methaemoglobin levels also interfere with the accuracy of the $SpO_2$ readings, which tend to read 85%, regardless of the actual $SaO_2$.
- Strong ambient light can contaminate the signal from the probe, though most machines can now compensate for this effect.
- Nail varnish can make it difficult for an accurate waveform to be detected. Long finger nails can impede positioning of the probe on the finger.
- Pressure injury can result from incorrect positioning or prolonged attachment of the probe. Burns have been reported with probes that are incompatible with the oximeter or with inadequately protected probes in the high magnetic fields found in MRI scanners.

# End-tidal $CO_2$ monitoring (capnography)

*Background theory*

Capnography is the technique of displaying the carbon dioxide ($CO_2$) levels in the airway during the respiratory cycle. During the first part of expiration, dead space gas from the airway (endotracheal tube, trachea, bronchi, and bronchioles down to, but not including, the respiratory bronchioles and alveoli) is exhaled first, leaving without exchanging any $CO_2$ with the blood in the lungs. The $CO_2$ signal then rises to a plateau as the gas containing $CO_2$ from the alveoli and respiratory bronchioles is exhaled. In healthy individuals, the $CO_2$ level at the end of expiration ($PE'CO_2$) approximates to the arterial partial pressure of $CO_2$ ($PaCO_2$).

The capnometer provides invaluable supplementary evidence that the endotracheal tube is in the correct position. If the tube has become dislodged into the oesophagus, it registers no or minimal $CO_2$. It can also be used to monitor respiratory rate and serves to indicate when a circuit disconnection has occurred.

Carbon dioxide absorbs infrared radiation. The $CO_2$ level in the respiratory gas is measured by comparing how much is absorbed in a sampling chamber with a known source. There are two types of capnometer: sidestream and mainstream. The former sucks gas from the airway circuit through a fine bore tube via a water trap and the sample is analysed within the machine itself. The latter's sensor is situated within the airway circuit. It does not require the energy expenditure to suck up the gases but needs an electrical supply to the sensor itself. As a result, the mainstream sensor tends to be bulkier and more vulnerable to damage.

*Set up procedure*

The capnometer should be set up and calibrated at regular intervals according to the manufacturer's instructions, but the following general principles may be helpful.

- Check that the sensor holder of a mainstream capnometer is patent and that the sensor panels are clean and not cracked.
- Visually check the sampling tubing of a sidestream sensor and ensure that the water trap is not full.
- Switch on and allow a warm up time with sensors attached to the breathing circuit.
- Ensure that the sensor or sampling tube is not lying dependently, so as to reduce the risk of secretions or condensation contaminating the sensor or blocking the tubing.
- Position the sensor or sampling tube to avoid traction on the endotracheal tube.
- Ensure that all airway connections are secure.

*Clinical problems*

- In ill or injured patients and in those receiving high levels of sedation or anaesthesia, the end-tidal $CO_2$ level may not reflect the arterial level. In such situations, there may be regional abnormalities in ventilation of the alveoli with inspired gas and their perfusion with circulating blood. If parts of the lung are well ventilated but poorly perfused, there can be significant differences between the $PE'CO_2$ and the $PaCO_2$. Expired gas from the poorly perfused areas receives little $CO_2$ from the blood and dilutes the $CO_2$ from well perfused areas as the expired gas mixes. This causes the $PE'CO_2$ to underrepresent the arterial value. This is particularly important when controlling levels in severe head injury. It is important to compare the $PE'CO_2$ with the $PaCO_2$ from a simultaneous arterial sample before setting off on a transfer.
- A high $PE'CO_2$ generally indicates underventilation, which may relate to a problem with the ventilator or to partial airway obstruction. If it is due to a ventilator circuit problem resulting in rebreathing of $CO_2$, this will be shown by an increase in the inspired $CO_2$ ($PiCO_2$). While a low $PE'CO_2$ may indicate excessive ventilation, caution must be exercised because of ventilation–perfusion mismatch, as explained above. Particular causes of a low $PE'CO_2$ include pulmonary embolism and shock states, resulting from hypovolaemia, sepsis or heart failure.
- The expired $CO_2$ waveform may provide clues to clinical or technical problems. In airway obstruction, it may continue to slope upwards during late expiration. If the patient is attempting to breathe on a portable ventilator, this may be revealed by dips on the plateau of the waveform. Excessive damping or flattening of the waveform may indicate blockage of the suction tubing in a sidestream capnometer. Contamination of a mainstream sensor by secretions, on the other hand, may cause the $PE'CO_2$ to be overestimated.
- If the function of the capnometer is in doubt, test it yourself by exhaling into the sampling port to confirm a normal waveform with an expected $PE'CO_2$ of 38–42 mmHg (5.0–5.6 kPa).

- High respiratory rates ($>30\,min^{-1}$) may preclude accurate measurement of $PE'CO_2$, especially in sidestream capnometers. As in pulse oximetry, the waveform serves as a quality control signal on which to judge the reliability of the readings.
- The fall in barometric pressure at altitude can result in an underestimate of $PE'CO_2$, unless the machine has a built-in altimeter to make corrections.

## Invasive pressure monitoring

### Background theory

Arterial pressure may be conveniently measured on a beat to beat basis using an intra-arterial cannula attached to a transducer by a fluid column. The transducer converts the pressure wave into an electrical signal, which is amplified and displayed by the monitor. The radial artery is the preferred site for the cannula, though femoral, dorsalis pedis, posterior tibial, and brachial sites are possible alternatives. A continuous flushing system, provided by a bag of heparinised saline pressurised to about 300 mmHg, channelled through a constriction, keeps the system patent. In addition, a mechanical flush device allows the clinician to clear the cannula and tubing manually.

As with the pulse oximeter and capnometer, the displayed waveform contains invaluable information and serves as a quality check, helping to identify both clinical and technical problems.

### Set up procedure

- A flush system should be prepared using heparinised saline ($1000\,UI^{-1}$).
- The tubing should be short ($<4$ feet) and non-compliant and the number of three-way taps minimised, so as not to distort the waveform.
- Ensure that all connections are tight, that there are no bubbles within the system, and that the flush bag is pressurised.
- Connect the indwelling cannula to the tubing and flush manually. Check the arterial waveform.
- Secure the transducer at the level of the fourth intercostal space in the midaxillary line.
- Zero the transducer according to the monitor's instructions, with the three-way tap open to atmosphere and to the transducer. Return the three-way tap to the in-line position to display the waveform and readings.

### Clinical problems

- An adequate blood pressure *per se* does not indicate tissue perfusion. Do not rely on such readings in isolation.
- The waveform may indicate clinical problems; a spiky waveform with a short systolic time or a marked respiratory swing may be seen in hypovolaemia.
- The waveform may also reveal technical problems, such as a resonant, overshooting trace or a flattened, overdamped trace. It is worth rechecking for bubbles and leaks, checking that the flush bag is still pressurised and flushing the line manually. Consider removing any unnecessary three-way taps or excessive tubing.
- Consider re-zeroing and comparing the readings with non-invasive blood pressure values in the event of unexpected values, but do not simply ascribe abnormalities to monitor dysfunction. It is more likely that the fault is with the patient, who may need urgent attention. Re-zero periodically during prolonged transfers.
- Because of the risk of damage to a pulmonary arteriole by a continuously "wedged" pulmonary artery balloon flotation catheter (Swan Ganz™) it is recommended that such catheters are withdrawn 5–10 cm before transportation.

## MUMMY WRAP

The mummy wrap (see Figure 8.9) is a simple and very neat way to prepare your patient for transfer. It prevents significant heat loss and also avoids trailing monitor leads and drug lines.

- Place the blanket or quilt beneath the patient by log rolling.
- Slide onto the board.
- Thread the monitor lead bundle out over the feet and hold the main line out of the way.
- Check all the lines and transducers are secure.
- Fold the quilt around the patient from each side.
- Fasten all the securing straps, leaving the edges of the quilt accessible along the midline of the patient.
- Wrap the head in a towel or other insulator.

Once wrapped, the patient should not have to be exposed again, as the main fluid line, your IV access, and the pumps are outside the wrap. Everything else is tidily hidden away inside the quilt.

An alternative to a quilt is a sleeping bag. Many of these incorporate a hood to prevent heat loss from the head.

**A – AIRWAY**

Need to establish definitive airway.
As a guide GCS <9

**IF IN DOUBT INTUBATE**

Consider:
- type of ETT
- nasal/oral
- method of securing
- differences in children
- cuff problems
- sedation/paralysis

**B – BREATHING**

Spontaneous – high flow oxygen,
non-rebreathing mask, sat up

Ventilated – set ventilator,
calculate oxygen requirement
? hyperventilation

Monitor $SaO_2$, $EtCO_2$, alarms,
contents gauge

**IMMOBILISATION**

**SPINAL BOARD**
– any suspicion of spinal injury,
then use the board

**SPLINTS/TRACTION**
– all fractures must be immobilised,
but splints can be cumbersome

**DEDICATED STRETCHERS**
– for use in aircraft, mountain
rescue extrication, etc.

**EYES**

Do not forget to protect
the eyes during transport.

Remember that you may
need to regularly review pupil

**CERVICAL SPINE**

Any suspected Cx spine injury
requires formal immobilisation

Hard collar, headblocks and tape

Even without neck injury, it is
often useful to stabilise the head
for fast transports (esp. children).

e.g. upturned receivers + tape

**C – CARDIOVASCULAR**

Few indications to move patient
before stable

Monitor ECG, NIBP/IBP, CVP,
PA, urine, temperature

Bundle monitor leads together

Fasten transducers to upper arms
to be readily accessible

Two large bore cannulae, blood
set attached to main line

Avoid infusion pumps, rationalise
all infusions. Use syringe driver
whenever possible (check batteries)

Keep one route of venous access
easily to hand, outside the wrap

**"MUMMY WRAP"**

Wrap the patient in an insulating blanket
or quilt from head to toe

- Reduces heat loss
- Avoids trailing limbs and leads
- Makes patient handling much easier

*Remember to keep one line for
IV access outside the wrap*

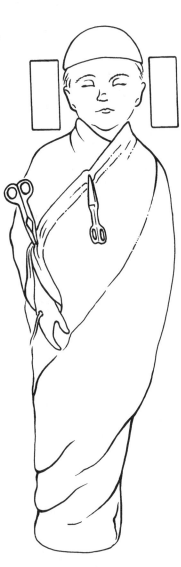

**Figure 8.9.** The mummy wrap.

# CHAPTER

# 9

# Communications: radio use and voice procedure

---

**Objectives**

- Understand the principles and practice of voice procedure.

---

## VOICE PROCEDURE

### Principles

The fundamentals of a good radio message are:

- clarity
- accuracy
- brevity.

Clarity can be achieved by attention to the voice's:

- rhythm
- speed
- volume
- pitch.

**Remember**: *RSVP*. The *rhythm* should be steady; the *speed* should be slightly slower than normal speech; for adequate *volume* it is not necessary to shout but do not whisper unless the radio has a specific whisper mode; the best *pitch* is that of a female voice and men with a gruff voice should make a conscious effort to raise their pitch.

To achieve *accuracy* and *brevity* requires discipline and practice. Air time is a valuable commodity. The system of radio voice procedure taught in this book is based on military voice procedure. Examples of alternative systems are given where appropriate.

# RADIO SHORTHAND

## Glossary

Brevity can be facilitated by using a number of special words, that act as a verbal shorthand. These are shown in Box 9.1.

---

**Box 9.1.   Special words used in radio voice procedure**

| | |
|---|---|
| Over | The speaker now wishes the receiver to talk |
| Out | The conversation is finished |
| Ok | I understand |
| Roger | I understand |
| Go ahead | I am ready to receive your message |
| Send | I am ready to receive your message |
| Acknowledge | Tell me you have received my message |
| Say again | Repeat what you said |
| ETA | Estimated time of arrival |
| ETD | Estimated time of departure |
| Wait | I cannot reply within the next 5 seconds (may be repeated once after 5 seconds, then WAIT OUT after further 5 seconds) |
| Wait out | I cannot reply, I will contact you later |
| Standby | Stay alert, further information to follow |

---

Other words may be in use locally. If so, it is essential that their full meaning is known and understood by all users of the net.

The following terminology is *not* acceptable:

- over and out – it is either over *or* out
- rodger dodger – slang
- ten four – slang.

It is not acceptable to swear on the radio.

## The phonetic alphabet

Difficult or important words should be spelt to avoid confusion. Rather than saying "Ay, Bee, See, Dee", a phonetic alphabet is used to give each letter a distinct sound: "Alpha, Bravo, Charlie, Delta…". These are shown in Box 9.2

---

**Box 9.2.   The phonetic alphabet**

| | | | |
|---|---|---|---|
| A | Alpha | G | Golf |
| B | Bravo | H | Hotel |
| C | Charlie | I | India |
| D | Delta | J | Juliet |
| E | Echo | K | Kilo |
| F | Foxtrot | L | Lima |

---

| M | Mike | T | Tango |
|---|------|---|-------|
| N | November | U | Uniform |
| O | Oscar | V | Victor |
| P | Papa | W | Whisky |
| Q | Quebec | X | X-ray |
| R | Romeo | Y | Yankee |
| S | Sierra | Z | Zulu |

**Example**

Mike One. Send further supply of oxygen, spell **O**scar-**X**-ray-**Y**ankee-**G**olf-**E**cho-**N**ovember. Acknowledge, over.

## Numbers and figures

For accuracy, the pronunciation of numbers is stressed, as shown in Box 9.3.

**Box 9.3.   Number pronunciation**

| | |
|---|------|
| 1 | wun |
| 2 | too |
| 3 | thuree |
| 4 | fower |
| 5 | fiyiv |
| 6 | six |
| 7 | seven |
| 8 | ate |
| 9 | niner |
| 0 | zero |

**Example**

Mike One. I require two hundred and fifty, figures too-fiyiv-zero, milligrams of cefotaxime, over.

## BASIC MESSAGE HANDLING

### Initiating a call

1. To start a message, say "hello" to the station being called.
2. Next state who you are.
3. Finish the message with "over" (to indicate that the other station can now speak).

**Example**

Hello Control, this is Mike One, over.

It is also acceptable to initiate a message in the following way:

> **Example**
>
> Mike One to Control, over.
> Control from Mike One, over.

## Replying to a call

Prefix each message with the call sign of the station sending the message.

> **Example**
>
> Control. Go ahead, over.
> Mike One. Send another ambulance.

## Replying to a group call

Occasionally Control or another station will call all the stations on the net. Replies should be in alphanumerical order. Each station is allowed five seconds during which to reply. After this time the next station should reply.

> **Example**
>
> Hello all stations, this is Control. Acknowledge my last message, over.
> Mike One. Acknowledged, over.
> Mike Two. Acknowledged, over.
> 5 SECOND PAUSE
> Mike Four. Acknowledged, over.
> Control. Mike One, Two, and Four acknowledged. Out.

## Ending a call

Finish a message with "out". Only one user needs to say "out".

> **Example**
>
> Control, OK, over.
> Mike One, out.

Ambulance Control in some areas may always wish to have the last word and the following unnecessary transmission will occur after the messages shown above:

> Control, base out.

## Offering a message

Theoretically on a constantly monitored radio net it should not be necessary to "offer" a message. That is to say, you should be able to move straight into the text of the message. However, experience shows that messages *do* need to be offered as the recipient is not always fully alert and may not be in a position to write things down.

1. Initiate the message as shown above.
2. Before finishing indicate that a message is to be sent.
3. Finish the message with "over" as before.

> **Example**
>
> Hello Control, this is Mike One. Message, over.

# ADVANCED MESSAGE HANDLING

## Corrections

From time to time you will make errors when sending a message. These errors must be corrected. To correct a message:

1. as soon as an error has been made, say "wrong"
2. follow this with the correct message
3. if necessary, repeat the message for clarity.

> **Example**
>
> Mike One. I have now moved to grid thuree-too-wun wun-seven-six. Wrong. Grid thuree-too-wun *too*-seven six. I say again, thuree-too-wun too-seven-six, over.

## Repeating

On a military radio net the instruction "say again" is used for a message to be repeated; "repeat" is reserved for artillery to fire again! On a civilian net it is acceptable to say "repeat". To have a message repeated:

1. as soon as the message ends (the sender says "over"), reply as shown above
2. ask for the message to be repeated or said again
3. finish the message with "over" as before.

> **Example**
>
> Mike One. Say again, over

If only part of a message need be repeated, then specify which part as shown in Box 9.4.

---

**Box 9.4.  Repeating part of a message**

"Say again all after…" Repeat everything after the specified word.
"Say again all before…" Repeat everything before the specified word.
"Say again all between…" Repeat everything between the specified words.

---

**Example**

Mike One. Say again all between PRIORITY and AMBULANCE, over.

---

## Long messages

Occasionally it is necessary to send a long message on the radio. This should be broken down into a series of shorter messages and the receiver should be asked to acknowledge that they have received each part. Not only does this ensure accuracy but it gives the opportunity for others on the net to interrupt if they have a more urgent message. Some radios are programmed to stop transmission after a time (e.g. 20–30 seconds). Most Ambulance Service systems are not programmed in this way yet. To send a long message:

1. offer a message as shown above
2. before finishing, indicate that a "long message" is to be sent
3. at frequent intervals (never longer than 30 seconds) ask the receiving station to "acknowledge so far"
4. repeat any part of the message not received
5. when certain that the message that has been sent already has been correctly received, send the next part of the message
6. repeat steps 3–5 until all the message has been sent
7. finish the message.

---

**Example**

Hello Control, this is Mike One, long message, over.
Control. Go ahead, over.
Mike One. Require *wun* doctor and nurse team and *too* paramedics to move severely injured patients now, acknowledge so far, over.
Control. Roger so far, over.
Mike One. Team to take twenty, figures *too-zero*, bottles of Haemaccel, spell **H**otel-**A**lpha-**E**cho-**M**ike-**A**lpha-**C**harlie-**C**harlie-**E**cho-**L**ima, acknowledge, over.
Control. Team to take figures too-zero bottles of Haemaccel, over.
Mike One. Yes. Out.

---

## Relaying a message

If all mobiles are not in contact with Control it is sometimes necessary for messages to be passed to one station via another. It is essential that all stages of this process are accurate.

1. The initiator of the message offers a message to an intermediary as shown above.
2. Before finishing the initiator indicates that the message is to be passed to another call sign (the final recipient).

3. The message is passed to the intermediary.
4. The intermediary acknowledges the message and ends the call with the initiator.
5. The intermediary offers a message to the final recipient.
6. Before finishing the intermediary indicates that the message is being passed from the initiator.
7. The message is passed to the final recipient.
8. The intermediary ends the call to the final recipient.
9. The intermediary calls the initiator and indicates that the message has been passed.

---

**Example**

Hello Mike One, this is Control. Message for Mike Four, over.

Mike One. Send, over.

Control. Message for Mike Four. Send two drug packs to the road, over.

Mike One. Roger out to you. Hello Mike Four, this is Mike One, message from Control, over.

Mike Four. Send, over.

Mike One. From Control, send two drug packs to the road, over.

Mike Four. Roger, over.

Mike One. Out to you. Hello Control, this is Mike One. Message passed, over.

Control. Roger, out.

---

# THE RADIO CHECK AND SIGNAL STRENGTH

It is important that all stations on any net, and particularly Control, know how good communications are. This is achieved using the *radio check*. Radio checks can be initiated by Control or by other call signs. To perform a radio check:

1. initiate call to the station or group of stations to be checked
2. before finishing indicate that a "radio check" is being performed
3. finish the message with "over"
4. await the replies
5. indicate the results of the check to the station or group of stations
6. end the call.

---

**Example**

Hello Control, this is Mike One, radio check, over.
Control. OK, over.
Mike One. OK, out.

---

If communications are not OK then they can be classified as:

| | |
|---|---|
| **Difficult** | Most words are heard but there is interference. |
| **Broken** | Messages are heard intermittently. |
| **Unworkable** | Only occasional words are heard – or interference only. |
| **Nothing heard** | Nothing is heard at all. |

# CHAPTER 10

# Moving and handling

---

**Objectives**

- Discuss the general principles of Health and Safety.
- Discuss the principles of moving and handling.

---

## GENERAL LEGISLATION

The UK legislation which governs all aspects of safety in the workplace is encompassed in the Health and Safety at Work Act 1974 and any subsequent amendments and additions.

The Act is overseen by the Health and Safety Executive (HSE). The HSE's mission statement is: "To ensure that risks to people's health and safety from work activities are properly controlled".

Increasingly, UK agencies such as the HSE are working with mainland European partners, in the European Committee for Standardisation (CEN). The CEN's mission is to promote voluntary technical harmonisation in Europe. European Standards are developed on the basis of voluntary agreement between all the interested parties. Once a member state has agreed the standard, this is likely to become law.

The Health and Safety legislation covers all aspects of safety in the workplace and in the context of transfer medicine, specifically:

- manual handling
- reporting of incidents
- equipment safety
- vehicle design and safety
- handling of clinical waste.

## THE LAW AND MANUAL HANDLING

The Manual Handling Operations Regulations (1992) state that when faced with a hazardous manual handling activity, the following hierarchy should be adhered to.

1. **Avoidance** – if reasonably practical.
2. **Automation** – if reasonably practical, the whole or part of the process.
3. **Assessment** – risks must be assessed.
4. **Reduction** – identified risks should be reduced to their lowest level.
5. **Review** – to ensure additional risks are not created and to monitor the effectiveness of risk reduction techniques.

## Avoidance

Avoid unnecessary movement.

## Automation

**Trusts are obliged to provide appropriate moving and handling equipment**. Hoists should be used where provided but Patslides™ may be used as an alternative. Hydraulic assisted ambulance stretchers should be used when possible and ambulance vehicles with ramp entrance are recommended. The CEN is developing new standards for ambulances which address these issues, amongst others.

## Assessment

The Manual Handling Operations Regulations require the assessment of risks surrounding hazardous manual handling activities. A risk assessment increases awareness and therefore should reduce accidents. If something were to go wrong, the risk assessment would be used as evidence. All individuals exposed to the risk should be identified and they should have access to the risk assessment.
**Risk assessment should address what actually happens, <u>not what should happen</u>**.
Risk assessment in general considers the risks associated with:

- the task
- the individual
- the load
- the environment

For each of the following movements a risk assessment and plan should be formulated for:

- transfer between bed/trolley to ambulance stretcher
- adjusting the height of the stretcher
- wheeling the stretcher
- moving into and out of the ambulance
- transfer between ambulance stretcher to bed.

## Reduction

Identified risks should be reduced to their lowest level using knowledge about the forces used in moving and handling operations.

- Knowing how to apply the principles of leverage.
- Knowing how to use knowledge about your own and the load's centre of gravity.

- Knowing how to apply forces, which muscle groups to use, and the effects of momentum.
- Knowing how to reduce friction.

## Review

There should be an ongoing review of the tasks involved in moving and handling that takes into account currently available equipment.

## SAFETY PRINCIPLES OF HUMAN MOVEMENT APPLIED TO MANUAL HANDLING

Despite adequate risk assessment, there will still be times when the patient movement must be undertaken manually.

**Remember**: any manual handling operation involving the movement of patients is a potentially hazardous risk.

Incorrect manual moving and handling techniques can damage your back. Avoid the following:

- bending
- stooping
- overloading
- twisting
- maintaining a fixed posture.

The same techniques which are used for manual handling of patients can be applied to moving and lifting stretchers, heavy or bulky equipment or stores.

## Plan the move

Prepare the environment, load, and equipment. This includes appropriate footwear to provide a good grip to ensure a stable platform.

Make sure one of you (agreed in advance) gives the instructions and explains to colleagues (and the patient if he is aware) exactly what you are going to do: "We'll move halfway across after the count of three … one … two … three … move".

## Getting ready to move

The centre of gravity in normal adults (when standing) is just in front of and near the base of the spine.

Maintain a stable base. Feet should be placed shoulder width apart; when standing with feet together, the base area is only the size of a pair of shoes and a little pressure from the side will cause the body to fall or sway. To remain upright and to stop you falling backwards or forwards, place one foot in front of the other with the back foot pointing outwards.

Keep the centre of gravity of the load as close as possible to your own centre of gravity.

## Executing the move

- Relax, avoid tensing your muscles, keep the spine in a natural position, and your knees soft.
- Communicate with others involved.
- Establish a firm grip on the load.
- Lead the movement with your head.
- Power the move with major muscle groups: legs, and buttocks.
- Avoid bending; move your feet, not your trunk.

## Lifting

Some staff still talk in terms of "lifting and handling…"; however, lifting should be avoided whenever possible. If, after a risk assessment, there is no alternative to lifting then:

- keep your back straight – a straight spine is in the least danger
- bend your knees and hips – use the leg muscles, they are the strongest in the body
- keep your chin tucked in
- make sure your grip is no wider than the width of your shoulders
- stand with your feet apart (allowing a balanced distribution of your weight)
- stand close to the object or patient being lifted
- hold the load as close to your body as possible
- tuck your elbows well in
- use your body weight to counterbalance the load
- when you can get the load moving, often it will follow through under its own momentum
- break the lifting down into stages; this will give you a rest between efforts
- when using lifting equipment, make sure you use it correctly.

## Using a Patslide™

- Ensure adequate number of personnel:
  - to protect airway and neck
  - either side of patient
  - per leg splint (if present).
- Transfer coordinated by person managing the airway.
- Warn patient.
- Slight rotation of patient, insert Patslide™ under sheet.
- Check that no line or tube is likely to be snared in the move.
- Slide over.
- Remove Patslide™.

**Summary**

Understanding the principles of manual handling will enable you to make a risk assessment, plan each movement and reduce the risk of injury.

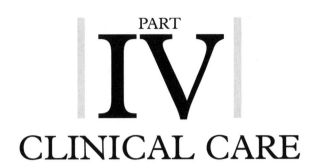

PART

IV

CLINICAL CARE

# 11

# General

**Objectives**

- To outline the general clinical approach to a patient requiring transfer.

## INTRODUCTION

Controlling the patient's care requires both a systematic examination and appropriate treatment to be carried out. A structured approach comprises:

- primary survey and resuscitation
- secondary survey and emergency treatment.

The aim of the primary survey is to identify and treat any immediately life threatening conditions. This differs from the traditional clinical teaching, i.e. taking a history from the patient followed by clinical examination, the reason being that such an approach can potentially delay implementing a life saving treatment.

The primary survey should be repeated frequently to detect any change in the patient's condition so that appropriate resuscitative measures can be commenced immediately.

Once any immediate life threatening conditions have been either treated or excluded, a comprehensive history can be taken and a thorough examination can be carried out. This is known as the secondary survey. During this phase emergency treatment should continue as necessary. By the end of the secondary survey a formal management plan must be developed. This needs to include consideration of whether the patient requires transportation to another facility.

# PRIMARY SURVEY AND RESUSCITATION

> During the primary survey, the aim is to **hunt out** and treat all **immediately life threatening** conditions.

Key components of the primary survey are:

- **A** – airway control (and spine immobilisation when appropriate)
- **B** – breathing
- **C** – circulation (and haemorrhage control when appropriate)
- **D** – disability
- **E** – exposure.

## A – airway control and spine immobilisation when appropriate

Aim:

- clear and secure the airway
- administer oxygen
- maintain spine immobilisation in appropriate cases.

You must initially assume the presence of spinal instability if the patient is a victim of blunt trauma or if the mechanism of injury indicates this region may have been damaged. In such patients, none of the activities used to clear and secure the airway must involve movement of the neck. You should manually immobilise the cervical spine at the same time as talking to the patient. This not only establishes supportive contact but also can be used to assess the airway.

If the patient responds appropriately the airway can be considered to be patent, breathing is occurring, and there is adequate cerebral perfusion. If no answer is forthcoming then chin lift or jaw thrust manoeuvres must be carried out to prevent the tongue obstructing the patient's upper airway. The patency of the airway is reassessed by:

- **looking** – for chest movement
- **listening** – for the sounds of breathing
- **feeling** – for expired air.

A rapid assessment for other causes of airway obstruction should include inspection for vomit, trauma, foreign bodies, macroglossia, and stridor.

When a chin lift or jaw thrust is needed, then an airway adjunct may be required to maintain patency. A nasopharyngeal airway is useful in the conscious patient, but is contraindicated if there are signs indicative of a base of skull fracture. Patients with an impaired gag reflex usually benefit from an oropharyngeal airway. A decision must then be taken on the need for intubation to either maintain the airway or provide adequate oxygenation. Rarely is a surgical airway required.

Once definitive control of the airway has been achieved, supplemental oxygen should be given to all patients who have respiratory difficulty or who are bleeding. If the patient is not intubated, oxygen should be delivered, ideally using a non-rebreathing mask and reservoir. This enables the fractional inspired oxygen ($FiO_2$) to reach a level of approximately 0.85. Even patients who have chronic air flow limitation (e.g. chronic bronchitis/emphysema) should receive high flow oxygen initially. This can subsequently be reduced according to its clinical effect and arterial blood gas results.

The neck should then be inspected quickly for:

- swellings and wounds which can indicate there is local injury or damaged blood vessels
- subcutaneous emphysema from a pneumothorax or mediastinal emphysema
- tracheal deviation suggesting a tension pneumothorax
- tracheal tugging suggesting respiratory difficulty
- distended neck veins indicating there is a rise in the central venous pressure from a tension pneumothorax, cardiac tamponade or damage to the great vessels
- laryngeal crepitus indicating a fracture of the laryngeal cartilage.

## B – breathing

Aim:

- detect and treat life threatening respiratory conditions.

---

**Box 11.1.  Life threatening respiratory conditions**

- Tension pneumothorax
- Open chest wound
- Flail chest
- Life threatening bronchospasm

---

A patent airway does not ensure adequate ventilation. The latter requires an intact respiratory centre along with adequate pulmonary function augmented by the coordinated movement of the diaphragm and chest wall.

Examination should entail **inspection** for the presence of cyanosis, respiratory rate, and effort as determined by accessory muscle use, intercostal recession, and symmetry.

---

**Box 11.2.  Chest inspection**

- Marks/rash
- Rate
- Effort
- Symmetry

---

With respect to **palpation**, the position of the trachea and apex beat will detect any mediastinal shift. In cases of trauma, the sternum and each rib should be felt for tenderness, deformity, and overlying surgical emphysema.

The anterior chest wall must be **percussed** in the upper, middle, and lower zones assessing the difference in note between the two sides. This procedure needs to be repeated on the posterior chest wall and also in the axilla to detect areas of hyperresonance (air), dullness (interstitial fluid) or stony dullness (pleural fluid). In cases of possible spinal injury, the patient will need to be turned in a coordinated fashion. This is known as log rolling and can be delayed until the end of the secondary survey unless a posterior penetrating wound is suspected. **Auscultation** can then be performed to establish whether breath sounds are either absent, present or masked by added sounds.

Further information regarding the patient's respiratory state will be obtained by attaching them to a pulse oximeter.

*Tension pneumothorax*

> **Box 11.3.   Signs of a tension pneumothorax**
>
> - Tachypnoea
> - Hypotension
> - Hyperresonant hemithorax
> - Decreased air entry to the hemithorax
> - Deviated trachea (late)
> - Raised JVP (if no hypovolaemia)
> - Cyanosis (very late)

In a short period of time these patients become shocked as cardiac output falls and ventilation becomes progressively more difficult as the intrapleural pressure increases. This may be noticed in patients who are being ventilated, either as increasing resistance to manual ventilation or raised inflation pressures.

A raised JVP will only occur if there is sufficient blood volume. Cyanosis is a late sign and depends on there being more than 5 g of deoxygenated (reduced) haemoglobin in the circulation.

In the trauma or unconscious patient a tension pneumothorax can be missed and so a high index of suspicion is required. It can also occur at any point in the resuscitation, especially after insertion of a central line or during positive ventilation where there are rib fractures.

The patient can die from this condition in the time it takes to obtain and process a chest radiograph. Therefore, as an emergency measure, a 16 G cannula connected to a 10 ml syringe is inserted into the second intercostal space in the mid-clavicular line. The aim is to decompress the chest. A rapid release of air confirms the diagnosis, following which the cannula can be slid over the needle into the pleural cavity and the syringe and needle removed. This procedure will give you enough time to definitively treat the condition by inserting a chest drain.

Once the chest drain is in position, the drainage must be monitored. Underwater seals are unsuitable for transfers.

If, after insertion of the cannula, there is only a slow release of air and froth, then the diagnosis remains in doubt. There is also now a risk that a pneumothorax has been created as a result of the needle puncturing the lung. This creates a simple pneumothorax which can be transformed into a tension pneumothorax, particularly if the patient is being ventilated. An urgent chest radiograph is therefore required. If this is not possible then it is safer to insert a chest drain. You also need to remember that the cause of shock still has to be found. A possible missed diagnosis is a cardiac tamponade.

*Open chest wound*

An open chest wound will automatically produce a pneumothorax on the same side. A particularly dangerous situation is when air can enter via the hole but not escape (the "sucking chest wound"). This gives rise to a tension pneumothorax, either because the wound acts as a one-way valve (due to its shape) or from an inappropriately applied dressing.

The immediate management of an open chest wound is to apply an Ashermann seal so that air can escape during expiration but not enter through the defect during inspiration. A chest drain should then be inserted via a freshly created hole, so that the pneumothorax can be drained. In the acute situation of a tension pneumothorax developing, any occluding dressing must be removed. This opens the wound and allows air to escape. The long term management of the majority of these patients is by definitive surgical closure.

## Flail chest

Examination of the chest wall will reveal crepitus, instability and, in the conscious patient, pain.

These patients must be managed in such a way that their hypoxia is corrected. Initially this is by high flow, warm, humidified oxygen and adequate fluid resuscitation during the primary survey.

Analgesia, by intercostal or epidural block, is given during the definitive management phase. A selected group of patients (Box 11.4) require a more aggressive approach to correct their hypoxia, namely intubation and ventilation, usually early on in the resuscitation. In all cases the arterial blood gases (ABG) need to be monitored frequently.

---

**Box 11.4.   Patients with a flail chest requiring artificial ventilation**

- Falling $PaO_2$ or $<50$ mmHg (6.6 kPa) on air
- $PaO_2$ $<80$ mmHg with supplemental $O_2$
- Rising $PaCO_2$ or $>45$ mmHg (6 kPa)
- Exhaustion
- Respiratory rate $>30$/min
- Significant associated injuries of the abdomen and head

---

## Life threatening bronchospasm

Life threatening bronchospasm and its effects can be recognised clinically (Box 11.5). It should be treated initially with a nebulised β2 agonist (e.g. salbutamol) and ipratropium bromide. This can then be followed by intravenous aminophylline (or salbutamol if already taking theophylline) and hydrocortisone.

---

**Box 11.5.   Life threatening bronchospasm**

- Silent chest
- Exhaustion
- Unable to complete sentences
- PEFR $<33$%
- Bradycardia
- Hypotension
- Decreased conscious level
- Normal or rising $PaCO_2$

---

Failure to respond with this therapy should lead you to consider intubation and ventilation at an early stage. An urgent chest radiograph will also be necessary to exclude a tension pneumothorax.

## C – circulation

Aim:

- detect and treat shock (i.e. inadequate delivery or utilisation of essential substrates by vital organs).

The circulatory phase of the primary survey consists of stemming any overt bleeding, assessment of the cardiovascular state, and managing shock.

Shock can result from vascular, cardiac, and tissue pathology acting separately or in combination to cause an inadequate delivery of oxygen to vital structures of the body:

- decrease in oxygen uptake by the lungs
- reduced venous return
- impaired cardiac function
- reduced arterial tone.

The first represents the "A" and "B" causes of shock and have been described previously. The "C" causes are described below.

*Reduced venous return*

This reduction in preload is commonly due to **hypovolaemia** or **interference with venous return**.

True hypovolaemia is associated with either blood or plasma loss. Upper gastrointestinal sources are a common cause for haemorrhage seen in medical patients. In contrast, excessive plasma loss is often seen at the extremes of age with gastroenteritis. In diabetic ketoacidosis, fluid loss is related to a combination of hyperventilation, osmotic diuresis, decreased body sodium, vomiting and, possibly, the precipitating condition.

The common causes impeding preload are shown in Box 11.6.

---

**Box 11.6.  Common interference causes of reduced preload**

- Massive pulmonary embolus
- Tension pneumothorax
- Cardiac tamponade
- High mean airway pressure (e.g. high PPV)
- Gravid uterus

---

Blood returning to the heart depends on the pressure gradient created by the high hydrostatic pressure in the peripheral veins and low hydrostatic pressure in the right atrium of the heart. Any reduction in this gradient, increasing right atrial pressure, will lead to a fall in venous return to the heart. External compression on the thorax or abdomen can have a similar action in obstructing the venous return. In the supine position, the gravid uterus can compress the inferior vena cava and impair venous return.

*Impaired cardiac function*

A variety of conditions can adversely influence ventricular function and lead to shock (Box 11.7).

> **Box 11.7. Summary of the cardiac causes of shock**
>
> | | |
> |---|---|
> | Endocardial | Acute valve lesion: |
> | | infective endocarditis |
> | | papillary muscle rupture |
> | Myocardial | Ventricular failure/conduction problems: |
> | | ischaemia/infarction |
> | | myocarditis |
> | | drugs |
> | | toxins |
> | Epicardial | Tamponade: |
> | | cardiomyopathy |

It is important to remember that antiarrhythmic drugs being taken by the patient, or administered acutely, may have a significant negative inotropic effect. The same effect is seen with certain drugs taken as an overdose, for example tricyclic antidepressants. Myocardial function can also be impaired by infection (myocarditis), an underlying cardiomyopathy or toxins associated with the systemic inflammatory response syndrome (SIRS) (see below). Cardiac tamponade, in addition to its effect on venous return, also impedes ventricular filling.

As can be seen from the description above, several factors can interfere with the effectiveness of the cardiac pump. However, the term cardiogenic shock is reserved for patients who have an impaired cardiac performance resulting from 40% or more of the ventricular myocardium being affected. Consequently shock due to hypovolaemia, vasovagal reactions, arrhythmias, and drug reactions must be excluded first.

*Reduced arterial tone*

*Anaphylactic shock* Anaphylaxis is due to an acute reaction to a foreign substance to which the patient has already been sensitised. This leads to a rapid degranulation of mast cells and basophils triggered by IgE. Anaphylactoid reactions have an identical clinical presentation but are not triggered by IgE and do not necessarily require previous exposure. Furthermore, they may not produce a reaction every time.

*Systemic inflammatory response syndrome and septic shock* It has long been recognised that the physiological and clinical signs of sepsis can result from a variety of causes as well as infection. As a consequence, the term systemic inflammatory response syndrome

> **Box 11.8. Recommended standard terminology**
>
> **SIRS**
>
> Resulting from a variety of severe causes, SIRS is manifested by two of the following:
>
> - temperature $>38°C$ or $<36°C$
> - heart rate $>90$/min
> - respiratory rate $>20$/min or $PaCO_2$ $<32$ mmHg (4.3 kPa)
> - WBC $>12\,000$ cell/mm$^3$, $<4000$ cell/mm$^3$ or $>10\%$ immature forms.
>
> **Sepsis**
>
> - SIRS resulting from documented infection.
>
> **Septic shock**
>
> Sepsis associated with organ dysfunction and SBP $<90$ mmHg (or a reduction of over 40 mmHg from baseline) in the absence of other causes for hypotension and despite adequate fluid resuscitation.

(SIRS) should be used when describing the inflammatory response and "Sepsis" should be reserved for SIRS patients with definite infection.

*Neurogenic shock*   A spinal lesion above T6 can impair the sympathetic nervous system outflow from the spinal cord below this level. As a consequence, both the reflex tachycardia and vasoconstriction responses to hypovolaemia are eliminated. The result is generalised vasodilation, bradycardia, and loss of temperature control. As neurogenic shock leads to a reduction in blood supply to the spinal column, it gives rise to additional nervous tissue damage.

## Management of the shocked patient

The treatment of shock consists of restoration of an adequate delivery of oxygen and not simply the restoration of a normal blood pressure.

---

**Key point**: It is important to remember that pain has an adverse effect on the patient's tolerance of shock, as it increases the tissue's oxygen requirements. Therefore every effort should be made to reduce the level of pain for both humanitarian and physiological reasons.

---

Start by identifying and treating any overt bleeding and then carry out a rapid assessment of the patient's haemodynamic status.

*Assessment*   A central pulse, ideally the carotid, should be assessed for rate, rhythm, and character. It is important, however, to compare both carotid pulses (not simultaneously) as a reduction or absence in one pulse may reflect focal atheroma or a dissecting aneurysm. The blood pressure should be taken and peripheral perfusion assessed using the capillary refill time. Finally, always check the patient's core temperature because this can have a marked effect on the patient's CVS state.

*Look* at the patient and note his or her colour as well as the presence of distended or flat neck veins, sweating, and distress. Then *feel* the pulse for either a brady or a tachycardia. Is the patient vasodilated with a bounding pulse? Then check the position of the apex beat if it is palpable. Finish by *listening* for the presence of a third sound and/or heart murmur/s.

Follow this cardiovascular assessment by connecting the patient to an ECG and BP monitor. Then obtain peripheral intravenous access with largest cannula possible (ideally a 14 or 16 G) and take 20 ml of blood for laboratory tests. These include FBC, U&E, glucose and, if clinically appropriate, crossmatch, cardiac enzymes, amylase, blood cultures, and toxicology.

The antecubital fossa is the site of choice for venous access. With hypovolaemia it is important that fluid is infused quickly so short, wide cannulae should be used because the flow of a liquid in a tube is inversely proportional to the length and directly related to its diameter. An arterial line should be inserted at the earliest opportunity and the blood gases measured.

If a peripheral site is not available in adults, central venous access is advocated. This procedure should **only** be done by experienced staff because of the potential for damaging the vein and neighbouring structures.

By the end of this assessment, the answers to the following questions should have been ascertained.

- Is shock present?
- If present, what is its likely cause?

## Hypovolaemic shock

In hypovolaemic shock the primary aim of treatment is to prevent further bleeding if at all possible. Examples of this include the use of a Sengstaken tube for a variceal bleed. Often, however, there is no definite source for blood or fluid loss. In these cases, the clinician should move onto the next stage of management which is assessing the degree of intravascular volume loss.

*Estimating volume loss and grading shock* The compensatory mechanisms evoked by "shock" are related to the decline in function of various organs. Thus by monitoring these changes it is possible to grade the degree of shock. Respiratory rate, capillary refill (see below), heart rate, blood pressure, urine output, and conscious level can be readily measured and so are important indicators of both the grade of shock and the response to treatment. These physiological changes can be used to divide hypovolaemic shock into four categories depending on the percentage blood loss. The important features are:

- a tachycardia often occurs early on due to the sympathetic response
- in Grade 2 shock the diastolic blood pressure rises, without any fall in the systolic component, leading to a narrowed pulse pressure. This is due to the vasoconstriction mediated by the compensatory sympathetic nervous system. Consequently, a narrow pulse pressure with a normal systolic blood pressure is an early sign of shock
- tachypnoea can indicate shock as well as underlying respiratory or metabolic pathology
- hypotension indicates a loss of approximately 30% of the circulating volume.

*Limitations to estimations of hypovolaemia* For some patients, blindly following the signs could lead to a gross over- or underestimation of the blood loss (Box 11.9). It is therefore important that management is based on the overall condition of the patient and not on isolated physiological parameters.

---

**Box 11.9. Pitfalls in assessing blood loss**

- Elderly
- Drugs
- Pacemaker
- Athlete
- Pregnancy
- Hypothermia
- Compensation
- Tissue damage

---

Once the degree of blood loss has been estimated, the clinician needs to consider the possible causes so that appropriate management can be introduced.

*General management* In Grade 1 shock, a litre of crystalloid is infused and the response monitored. If hypovolaemia is estimated to be Grade 2 or higher, 500 ml intravenous colloid challenge is required. The aim should be to maintain the haematocrit (packed cell volume) at 30–35% so that oxygen delivery is optimised. Red cell replacement is secondary, becoming more important with progressively larger blood losses.

All fluids given to patients need to be warmed before administration, to prevent iatrogenically induced hypothermia. A simple way of achieving this is to store a supply of colloids and crystalloids in a warming cabinet. This eliminates the need for warming coils during this phase of resuscitation, which increase resistance to flow and thereby slow the rate of fluid administration.

The above management should be modified in hypotensive patients where there is a definite bleeding source that has not been controlled. In these cases vigorous fluid resuscitation will lead to further bleeding and a worse prognosis. These patients require the origin of the bleeding to be controlled urgently. In the meantime fluid needs to be administered so that the blood pressure is maintained at 20 mmHg below the baseline. This is known as permissive hypotensive resuscitation.

*Cardiac tamponade*  As these patients are usually victims of penetrating trauma it is important to suspect this condition. The classic presentation of Beck's triad, pulsus paradoxus, and Kussmaul's sign is only seen in a third of trauma patients (Box 11.10). Muffled heart sounds, due to blood in the pericardium, are always difficult to hear. Typically the patient is shocked due to impaired filling of the left ventricle, but paradoxically has an elevated central venous pressure. This is due to impaired venous return to the right ventricle. However, time should not be wasted inserting a CVP monitor during the primary survey and resuscitation phase. Furthermore, coexisting hypovolaemia may prevent a rise in CVP.

---

**Box 11.10.   Signs of cardiac tamponade**

- Beck's triad:
  Shocked
  Raised JVP
  Decrease in heart sounds
- Pulsus paradoxus of > 10 mmHg
- Kussmaul's sign – raised JVP on inspiration

---

Temporary relief of the symptoms of cardiac tamponade can be gained by optimising venous return by increasing the rate of intravenous infusions and aspiration of the pericardial sac (pericardiocentesis). This latter procedure has significant risks and can be falsely negative in 25% of cases, usually because the blood has clotted. If blood is aspirated then the cannula can be left in the pericardial space and allowed to drain freely. This will delay the development of any recollection but in all cases a thoracotomy will be required for definitive care. In the conscious medical patient with tamponade, echocardiography should be used to facilitate needle pericardiocentesis. If this equipment is unavailable or the patient is deteriorating, then drainage of the pericardium should be done using ECG monitoring.

If the patient presents as a PEA arrest then resuscitation according to Advanced Life Support protocol is required augmented by pericardiocentesis.

*Arrhythmia*  Any rhythm disturbance causing haemodynamic instability needs to be identified at this stage and treated according to UK and European resuscitation guidelines.

*Massive pulmonary emboli*

These patients present in a shocked state, with marked dyspnoea, and may have a preceding history of a DVT. In addition, there can be chest pain, syncope, and occasionally haemoptysis. In view of the right outflow obstruction, right heart strain is usually evident on the ECG. Due to the ventilation–perfusion mismatch, the $PaO_2$ is invariably low. In addition, neurohumoral factors are released which cause pulmonary vasoconstriction and occasional wheezing. Some alveoli become overventilated compared to the perfusion. As a result the dead space increases and the expired $PCO_2$ falls. If a pulmonary artery occlusion catheter is inserted, a high right ventricular pressure will be recorded along with a low cardiac output.

Diagnosis is difficult and depends on a high index of suspicion and exclusion of other possible causes. Depending upon the clinical state of the patient, several investigations can be carried out (Box 11.11). However, when dealing with a moribund patient the clinician may have to base the immediate management solely on their clinical suspicion. In such situations carry out a 12 lead ECG and a CXR to quickly exclude other causes of cardiovascular collapse.

---

**Box 11.11. Investigations for diagnosing a PE**

- V/Q scan
- Colour flow Doppler of the lower limbs
- Arteriography
- D-dimer
- Spiral CT
- Transoesophageal echocardiography
- Thoracic impedance

---

*Management*   As with all shocked patients, the airway needs to be cleared and secured and high flow oxygen provided. Intravenous access should also be obtained and a fluid bolus of 500 cc of crystalloid provided to attempt to increase the perfusion pressure. Should this fail, consider using vasopressors to maintain the diastolic pressure and thereby help coronary artery perfusion. Once the diagnosis is made thrombolytics should be administered by a peripheral line provided there are no contraindications. This should then be followed by a heparin infusion. As 20% of patients with a massive PE re-embolise during lytic therapy, some authorities advocate insertion of a temporary vena caval umbrella.

*Impaired cardiac function*

Shock resulting from heart failure is common. If this is suspected, it is essential to discover the past medical history and current medications. Clinically, in addition to the more usual signs of shock, there may be evidence of left and/or right ventricular failure and/or a dysrhythmia. These are summarised in Box 11.12.

---

**Box 11.12. Signs of cardiogenic shock**

- Raised JVP
- Basal crepitations
- Third heart sound
- Occasionally marked dyspnoea and central cyanosis from pulmonary oedema
- Occasionally murmurs depending upon the cause of the cardiogenic shock

---

Patients with heart failure are less able to compensate for hypovolaemia, should that coexist. This problem is compounded by the fact that measurement of the CVP does not provide an accurate estimate of the left ventricular end diastolic pressure (Box 11.13). These patients are therefore best managed using a pulmonary artery catheter which enables both the filling pressure of the left side of the heart and the cardiac output to be estimated and accurate fluid resuscitation provided.

---

**Box 11.13.  Disadvantages of CVP monitoring in heart failure**

- Measuring right ventricular pressure
- Often raised due to lung pathology
- Affected by positive pressure ventilation
- Malpositions causing false elevations

---

*Management*   It has been demonstrated that the first management priority is correction of hypoxaemia, even if this requires intubating and ventilating the patient with supplemental oxygen. When cardiogenic shock is due to right heart failure, a test infusion of 200 ml of colloid should be administered and the effect assessed. In contrast, when filling pressures are high, these need to be reduced in a controlled fashion. Intravenous nitrates are often used as they lower the systemic vascular resistance. Dopamine and Dobutamine may also be required to provide inotropic support and improve the cardiac output. Any dysrhythmia causing haemodynamic compromise must also be treated.

It is not unusual to find that a combination of mechanical ventilation, vasodilators, inotropes, and fluids is required to increase the cardiac index and $DO_2$. Clearly these are not procedures to be undertaken in the emergency department or medical ward, but require the facilities available in CCU, HDU or ITU.

*Anaphylactic shock*

Clinical manifestations include:

A   Oedema of the face and tongue
    Laryngeal oedema
B   Bronchoconstriction
    Respiratory arrest
C   Myocardial infarction
    Cardiovascular collapse

In view of the variety of chemical mediators released, cardiovascular collapse can result from one or more of the following reasons:

- arrhythmia
- hypovolaemia
- decreased myocardial function
- pulmonary hypertension.

Arrhythmias may result from direct mediator effects as well as hypoxia, hypotension, acidosis, pre-existing cardiac disease, and epinephrine given during resuscitation. Hypovolaemia can occur very quickly, with up to 50% of the circulating plasma volume being lost within 10–15 minutes in severe cases. This is brought about by a combination of increased vascular permeability, vasodilation, and decreased venous return from raised intrathoracic pressure secondary to bronchospasm and positive pressure ventilation.

*Management*   The management of anaphylactic shock is dependent upon a rapid ABC assessment and resuscitation, considering the diagnosis and preventing any further absorption of the suspected causative agent. Beware that a careful watch is required because airway obstruction, bronchospasm, and hypotension can have a delayed presentation.

Resuscitation consists of the standard care with a colloid fluid bolus of 10–20 ml/kg IV and epinephrine. As the latter reverses all the effects of anaphylaxis it should be used in patients with airway compromise, bronchospasm or hypotension.

0.5 mg of epinephrine should be given IM under ECG control. This can then be repeated after five minutes if there has been a failure to respond.

The role of other drugs is secondary to the above management. There is no conclusive evidence that antihistamines and steroids help. However, glucagon may be useful if the patient is on β blockers and is resistant to epinephrine.

Following resuscitation, the patient should be admitted for 8–12 hours of monitoring to detect those cases which develop a protracted or biphasic response. The latter is more likely following oral antigen ingestion or when symptoms started over 30 minutes after exposure.

### SIRS and sepsis

The diagnosis of septic shock can be difficult. In comparison with other causes of shock, except anaphylactic, the physiological features are usually (but not always) high cardiac output and low systemic vascular resistance (Table 11.1). The classic signs are a wide pulse pressure and warm skin due to the dilated peripheral vessels, agitation, pyrexia, and an increased respiratory rate due to the hypoxia. Later on the classic features of hypovolaemic shock are manifested with peripheral vasoconstriction and a low or normal core temperature. There may also be evidence of disseminated intravascular coagulation. This abnormality often manifests as blood oozing around wounds and cannula sites.

**Table 11.1.** Haemodynamic variables in shock (adult mean values).

|  | LAP* (mmHg) | CO** (l/min) | SVR*** (dyn/s/cm$^2$) |
|---|---|---|---|
| Normal | 10 | 5 | 1200 |
| Left ventricular failure | 25 | 2 | 3000 |
| Haemorrhage | 0 | 3 | 3000 |
| Sepsis | 2 | 12 | 3000 |
| Anaphylaxis | 2 | 12 | 300 |

\* Left atrial pressure
\*\* Cardiac output
\*\*\* Systemic vascular resistance

The type of septic shock known as the toxic shock syndrome has many potential causes. However, the clinical presentation remains the same:

- temperature $>38.9°C$
- macular, blanchable rash
- hypotension
- evidence of involvement of at least three systems.

The rash can be localised or general and tends to lead to desquamation after 1–2 weeks in survivors. Common systems which are involved are gastrointestinal (diarrhoea and vomiting), neurological (confusion, drowsy), renal (impaired function), muscle (myalgia, high CPK), haematological (leucocytosis, DIC, thrombocytopenia).

> **Key points**
>
> - Maintain a high index of suspicion because diagnosing septic shock can be difficult.
> - Always check for the non-blanching purpuric rash of meningococcal septicaemia.
> - Consider the diagnosis in any ill patient with an altered conscious level and haemodynamic instability without any obvious cause.

*Management*  If these patients are to survive, the source of the infection needs to be removed. Repeated blood cultures are required to determine the causative organism. Antibiotic therapy should be aimed at the most likely organism. However, often a combination of a penicillin, aminoglycoside, and metronidazole is often used according to the hospital antibiotic policy. If meningococcal septicaemia is suspected give Ceftriaxone 2 g intravenously **immediately**. When there is a collection of pus, drainage will be required either surgically or percutaneously under imaging control.

The patient will require cardiovascular and respiratory support, as well as intensive monitoring of their fluid and antibiotic regimes. The former aims to maintain a high cardiac index (over 4.5 l/min/m$^2$), high $DO_2$ (above 600 ml/min/m$^2$) and tissue perfusion pressure. This usually entails intubating and ventilating the patient with supplemental oxygen, correction of hypovolaemia with colloid, and the use of inotropes.

The indications for ventilation are no different from those routinely used:

- inability to maintain an airway
- inability to maintain normal $PaO_2$ and $PaCO_2$
- persistent tachypnoea despite adequate oxygenation and volume replacement
- persistent metabolic acidaemia
- elevated serum lactate.

The response to all vasoactive drugs is unpredictable. It is therefore advisable to start with a low dose and titrate further amounts until the cardiac index is sufficient to allow acceptable tissue perfusion. In adults this is usually at a level greater than 4.5 l/min/m$^2$.

Norepinephrine is frequently needed for its $\alpha$ agonist activity which helps counteract some of the profound vasodilation.

*Neurogenic shock*

The effects of neurogenic shock result from the loss of sympathetic output. This gives rise to a SBP of approximately 90 mmHg with a heart rate of around 50/minute. In addition the patient has warm and pink skin due to vasodilation. However, due to an initial pressor response releasing catecholamines into the circulation, the onset of these signs can take minutes to hours to develop. This situation may persist for up to 24 hours before levels of catecholamines fall enough to reveal the neurogenic shock.

The lack of sympathetic tone decreases the patient's response to other types of shock. It also enhances the vagal effect produced by stimulation of the pharynx, for example during laryngoscopy. This can lead to profound bradycardia requiring treatment with glycopyrrolate. Atropine can be used but it produces dry, thick secretions which increase the lung dysfunction.

Due to the nature of the injury the patient will also present with motor and sensory loss. However, these are difficult to assess in the unconscious patient. If in doubt, immobilise the C-spine and request a neurosurgical/orthopaedic review.

> **Key points**
>
> - Beware of the unconscious patient who is admitted following a fall downstairs. The initial neurological features are often attributed to an underlying stroke.
> - Spinal stabilisation must be maintained until specialist advice is obtained if a spinal injury is suspected from either the mechanism of the injury or examination.

*Management*  These patients require their airway to be secured by intubation as the risks of regurgitation and aspiration are increased due to the presence of a paralytic ileus, a full stomach, and an incompetent gastro-oesophageal sphincter. As close as possible to 100% oxygen should be administered, not least because the damaged spinal cord is very sensitive to hypoxia. During these activities the spine must be immobilised. With respect to the neck this can be achieved by an assistant holding the head or by the use of commercially available apparatus.

> **Key point**: Intubation is not contraindicated in the presence of cervical spine injury.

Persistent signs or symptoms of shock must not be attributed to the presence of spinal cord injury, particularly if there is penetrating trauma. Treatment of any bleeding source is still relevant in cases of spinal injury because of the risks of hypoperfusion of the spinal cord. In the presence of an isolated spinal cord injury, a systolic blood pressure of 80–90 mmHg is initially acceptable and usually achieved with a fluid challenge of 0.5–1 litre. Patients with an enduring bradycardia of less than 50 beats per minute should be given atropine 0.5–1 mg intravenously, repeated if necessary until the heart rate is acceptable. If this fails, inotropes may be required but this will involve the use of invasive haemodynamic monitoring to ensure the patient does not develop pulmonary complications due to inappropriate fluid management.

Early insertion of an arterial line is necessary in these patients. This provides continuous, accurate BP recordings as well as facilitating repeated ABG sampling. It is important that these patients are neither under- nor overtransfused. The former leads to further spinal injury, the latter leads to pulmonary oedema. As CVP recording is unreliable a pulmonary artery catheter should be inserted as soon as possible.

The loss of vascular tone in patients with high spinal injuries causes them to be prone to postural hypotension. This can occur in tipping or lifting the patient suddenly, as well as turning the trolleys at speed. As a result there can be underperfusion of areas of the body and episodes of ventilation–perfusion mismatch. It is therefore essential that these potential problems are prevented by the careful and coordinated movement of these patients.

During the initial neurological assessment using AVPU or GCS, an asymmetrical weakness may become apparent as may a lack of response to peripheral stimulation. These should be noted and a definitive neurological examination performed in the secondary survey. Finally, remember to keep the patient covered by warm sheets and blankets. This not only avoids embarrassment but also prevents heat loss from vasodilation which occurs after high spinal injuries.

Following the primary assessment and resuscitation, specialist advice should be sought regarding investigations and further management. Following plain radiographs, CT scanning has become the mainstay for spinal cord injuries. Its axial slices and reconstructive capabilities give CT scanning the ability to visualise middle and posterior column fractures. In addition, the degree of canal compromise can be accurately determined to within 1 mm or less. However, plain CT does not demonstrate any intraspinal contents other than bone fragments. Contrast enhancement is required for this and CT has been superseded by MR scanning. This is now the investigation of choice where visualisation of the contents of the spinal canal is required and ligamentous or intervertebral disc damage is suspected. Resuscitation equipment must be MRI compatible.

Published work has shown the advantage of giving high doses of methyl prednisolone in the first 24 hours, after blunt spinal injury (Box 11.14). The reason for this improvement is not known but workers have postulated that it could be due to a decrease in lipid peroxidation, protein degradation or catabolic activity or increased impulse conduction by activation of ion pumps.

---

**Box 11.14.   The early use of methylprednisolone following blunt spinal injury**

- 30 mg/kg IV over 15 minutes immediately.
- Then 5.4 mg/kg/hr for 23 hours.

---

Following evaluation of the spinal cord injury by plain radiography, CT, and MR scanning, a decision as to the need for surgical stabilisation can be made more accurately. In the early hours of management following cervical spine injury sufficient protection of the nervous system can be provided by inline stabilisation and log rolling with the patient's neck fixed in a hard collar. With radiological control, skull traction can be applied using increasing weights as necessary to maintain alignment without overdistraction.

## D – disability (neurological examination)

Aim:

- carry out a rapid neurological assessment and begin treating any immediately life threatening neurological condition.

*Assessment*

A rapid evaluation of the nervous system is performed by checking the size of the pupils, their reaction to light and by assessing the patient's conscious level using the AVPU system or Glasgow Coma Score.

---

**A** = **A**lert
**V** = Responding to **V**erbal stimulus
**P** = Responding to **P**ain
**U** = **U**nresponsive

---

**In the presence of any neurological dysfunction an assessment of the serum glucose is mandatory.**

---

If a serum glucose result is not immediately available then a bedside glucose estimate should be performed (Glucometer™, BM stix™).

*Resuscitation*

In the unconscious patient it is vital that the airway is cleared and secured and supplemental oxygen given until further information is available and investigations are carried out.

Naloxone should be considered if a narcotic overdose is suspected in a patient with a reduced conscious level. Coma associated with hypoglycaemia requires treatment as described previously. If meningitis is suspected Ceftriaxone 2 g IV stat should be given. Prolonged fitting should be controlled; lorazepam is the initial drug of choice.

## E – exposure

Aim:

- gain adequate exposure of the patient whilst keeping him/her warm.

It is impossible to perform a comprehensive examination unless the patient is fully undressed. Nevertheless care must be taken to prevent hypothermia, especially in elderly patients and children. This is done by covering patients between examinations and using a warm air blanket and warm intravenous fluids.

## Monitoring

The shocked patient's vital signs should be continuously monitored (Box 11.15).

---

**Box 11.15.  Monitored vital signs in hypovolaemic patients**

- Respiratory rate
- Peripheral oxygen saturation
- Heart rate
- Blood pressure
- Pulse pressure
- Capillary refill
- Chest leads (ECG rhythm and waveform)
- Temperature (core and peripheral)
- Urinary output
- Glasgow Coma Scale

---

The effectiveness of resuscitation is indicated by an improvement in the patient's clinical status. It is therefore important that this is measured and recorded frequently.

---

**If the patient deteriorates at any stage the primary assessment must be repeated, starting with A.**

---

## SECONDARY SURVEY

During the secondary survey the aim is to find new features and corroborative evidence to support or refute the working diagnosis.

The key components are a detailed medical history, a full examination and appropriate investigations. These should be obtained once vital functions have been stabilised and life threatening conditions have been treated.

## History

Nearly all medical diagnoses are made after a good history has been obtained from the patient. Occasionally this information may not be available, for a variety of reasons, so facts should be sought from relatives, the patient's medical notes, the general practitioner, friends or even the police and ambulance service. A well "phrased" history is required; this also serves as a useful mnemonic to remember the key features.

**P**    Problem
**H**    History of presenting problem
**R**    Relevant medical history
**A**    Allergies
**S**    Systems review
**E**    Essential family and social history
**D**    Drugs

The history of the presenting problems is of paramount importance. A comprehensive systems review will ensure that significant, relevant information is not excluded. In addition, it will help to refine the physical examination so that it is focused on the relevant symptoms.

## Examination

The overall appearance of the patient "from the end of the bed" can provide a lot of useful information. You can remember these signs by recalling the seven Ps in Box 11.16.

---

**Box 11.16.   All the Ps**

- Posture
- Pigmentation
- Pallor
- Pattern of respiration
- Pulsations
- Pronunciation
- Perspiration

---

A thorough head to toe, front to back examination of the patient should then be carried out.

## Re-evaluation

The patient must be monitored to assess the effect of treatment and to detect any deterioration in their condition. If this occurs then re-evaluation of the primary survey is mandatory.

By the end of the secondary survey you should have a working diagnosis plus a list of appropriate investigations and treatment. This also needs to include the necessity for transferring the patient to another unit (Box 11.17).

**Box 11.17.  Need for transfer**

- Specialist treatment
- Specialist investigations
- ICU/HDU bed

**Summary**

When called to see a patient you must quickly assess the situation and determine who is in charge and why you have been called. Going on to take control of the patient's care requires a structured approach. This is best divided into two key phases.

## Primary survey and resuscitation

To identify and treat immediately life threatening problems.

**Assessment of:**

A    Airway + C-spine immobilisation (when appropriate)
B    Breathing
C    Circulation + haemorrhage control (when appropriate)
D    Disability
E    Exposure.

**Resuscitation by:**

- clearing and securing the airway
- oxygenation and ventilation
- intravenous access and shock therapy
- monitoring respiration rate, pulse, blood pressure, oxygen saturation, urinary output, pupillary response, and conscious level.

## Secondary survey and emergency treatment

To gain corroborative evidence for the primary diagnosis and to identify new features.

The comprehensive physical examination needs to include a general overview and a systematic head to toe, front to back assessment.

# 12

# Special situations

---

**Objectives**

- To discuss systematically a wide range of clinical conditions and illustrate how the ACCEPT method can be applied to the transfer of these patients.

---

## INTRODUCTION

Each day in the UK, a variety of seriously ill and injured patients are transported within or between hospitals. The systematic ACCEPT approach enables these movements to be carried out safely and effectively. In previous chapters the components of ACCEPT have been described. It is now important to consider the wide range of clinical problems requiring transfer and see how the principles of ACCEPT can be applied to them.

The patients will be considered in three categories: trauma, medical (including non-trauma surgical), and paediatric. Patients with severe head injuries constitute a common group for transfer and are used as an example of the ACCEPT principles in practice.

## TRAUMA TRANSFERS

In the UK, trauma care is still managed on a district basis with a typical catchment population of 250 000–500 000. Currently, most cases go to the closest hospital rather than travelling directly to the tertiary centres, with their specialist services, such as neurosurgery and cardiothoracic surgery. As a result, most district general hospitals receive patients with major injuries directly from the scene of the incident and secondary interhospital transfer is frequently needed. Trauma patients often require early definitive surgery to save life or minimise disability. This critical time dependence influences the urgency of transfer.

Within a regional trauma system, specific indications for interhospital transfer usually relate to the anatomical injury and the associated specialist service. The most common injuries needing transfer are listed in Box 12.1. By its very nature, trauma tends to affect multiple body parts and different physiological systems. As a result, any central trauma-receiving hospital should have the full range of specialties on site to allow direct, integrated care of the injuries.

---

**Box 12.1.   Reasons for transferring trauma patients**

1.  Severe head injury (to a neurosurgeon)
    - Requiring a neurosurgical operation
    - Requiring neurosurgical assessment or intensive neurological monitoring
2.  Suspected mediastinal injury (to a cardiothoracic surgeon)
    - Aortic tear
    - Tracheobronchial rupture
    - Ruptured oesophagus
3.  Burns (to a plastic surgeon or specialist burns unit)
    - Extent (surface area and depth)
    - Particular site (e.g. airway and flexures)
4.  Spinal injuries (to a spinal surgeon or regional spinal unit)
    - Unstable fracture
    - Spinal cord injury
5.  Limb and pelvic injuries (to an orthopaedic, vascular or plastic surgeon)
    - Pelvic (including acetabular) reconstruction
    - Vascular injuries
    - Open tibial fractures with extensive soft tissue injury
    - Severe injuries to the hand
6.  Severe maxillofacial injuries (to a maxillofacial or plastic surgeon)
7.  Liver injuries (to a specialist hepatobiliary surgeon or liver unit)
8.  Severely injured children (to a specialist paediatric surgeon or paediatric ICU)
    - Requiring specialist paediatric surgery
    - Requiring intensive care
9.  Severely injured patients (to a regional trauma team, intensivist, rehabilitation specialist or local specialist, respectively)
    - With multiple injuries, according to regional trauma system guidelines, where it has been agreed to centralise major trauma in a trauma centre
    - Requiring regional or supraregional intensive care techniques
    - Requiring rehabilitation
    - Requiring repatriation or treatment in their home area

---

## Transfer of severely head injured patients to a specialist neurosurgical centre

Head injuries are common, with approximately one million cases per year in the UK. Approximately 90% are discharged home after initial assessment, leaving about 125 000 cases per year to be admitted to hospital, mainly for observation. Of these, 4–5% will need to be transferred to a regional neurosurgical unit for an emergency operation.

Patients with severe head injuries are prone to deterioration during transfer if proper preparation is ignored. It is essential that hypoxia and hypotension are avoided at all costs both by treating their cause before transfer and by monitoring appropriately during transfer. Even if the head injury is an isolated injury, it cannot be managed as a single system problem. Cardiorespiratory control goes hand in hand with nervous system management.

Further aspects of head injury care are considered in a later section, in which the ACCEPT approach to providing safe transfer for these patients is described in detail.

## Transfer to a specialist cardiothoracic centre

Most serious chest injuries are managed conservatively. In general, continuing care can be carried out in the primary hospital, without the need for transfer. Most pneumothoraces and haemothoraces are managed with simple chest drains. Unless there is a large, continuing air leak from tracheobronchial rupture or serious, continuing bleeding ($>200$ ml/hr) from injury to the lung or pulmonary vessels, there will be little need for thoracotomy. Most intensive care units are capable of managing a significant flail chest or severe pulmonary contusion. On the other hand, if the local ICU has no free beds, then such cases will need to be transferred.

Pulmonary contusion often worsens over the first few hours, so that the transferring team may find that the oxygenation worsens and airway pressures rise en route despite optimal care. The transferring clinician will need to distinguish this condition from other causes of deterioration, such as pneumothorax, haemothorax or endotracheal tube dislodgement into the right main bronchus. Management en route is helped by a capable transport ventilator with the capability to add $5$–$10\,cmH_2O$ positive end-expiratory pressure (PEEP).

The commonest reason for transfer to a cardiothoracic surgical unit after injury is for investigation and management of mediastinal injuries. Such injuries are usually suspected from the plain chest radiograph appearance. Previously, these patients were transferred for an arch angiogram to confirm or exclude the diagnosis of a ruptured aorta. Spiral CT scanning with intravenous contrast now allows an experienced radiologist at the primary hospital to exclude a ruptured aorta with confidence, though arch angiograms may still be needed in equivocal cases or if the scan does not demonstrate the site of rupture well enough to plan definitive surgery. Alternative imaging modalities are emerging, allowing less invasive investigation. For example, transoesophageal echocardiography has been claimed to be more sensitive at demonstrating small tears of the proximal aorta than arch angiography.

Many patients with traumatic disruption of the aorta are clinically stable, yet the adventitial layer of the aorta may be the only thing preventing exsanguination, the intimal and medial layers having been torn in the accident. The problem in transferring a patient with a ruptured aorta is to control the cardiovascular system so as to avoid high blood pressure, which may dislodge a clot and cause catastrophic bleeding, at the same time maintaining adequate flow to vital organs. Intubation should be managed with great care so as to avoid surges in blood pressure. Curbing the blood pressure during transfer may occasionally require antihypertensive agents but before resorting to them, it is important to provide adequate analgesia (if the patient is awake) and generous analgesia and sedation (if the patient is already intubated and ventilated).

## Transfer of patients with major burns to a specialist burns unit

Small, uncomplicated burns are generally managed without the need for transfer. Burns affecting more than 20% of the body surface area in adults or more than 10% in children or the elderly will need transfer to a regional burns unit. Those with full thickness burns greater than 5% of the body surface area in any age group should also be transferred. In addition, chemical burns and burns complicated by inhalation injury or involving specific body areas, such as the face, eyes, ears, perineum, genitalia and the flexures overlying joints, will commonly need transfer.

Careful assessment and resuscitation are needed prior to transfer. The injuries may not be confined to the more obvious burns. For example, the patient may have been hit by debris in an explosion or have jumped from an upper storey window in a house fire. The possibility of carbon monoxide poisoning and inhalation injury should be considered, especially if the incident occurred in a confined space or if the conscious level is altered. The clinical features include headache, nausea, confusion, and coma. Carbon monoxide poisoning is confirmed by measuring the carboxyhaemoglobin level with a co-oximeter, though there may not be good relationship between carbon monoxide level and symptoms or outcome. The immediate management of carbon monoxide poisoning is to administer 100% oxygen and to consider urgent transfer to a hyperbaric oxygen unit.

Inhalation injury is suggested by perioral burns, singed eyebrows or nasal hair, soot in the mouth or in sputum, pharyngeal erythema, hoarseness, stridor or by the need for high inspired oxygen concentrations to maintain the arterial saturation. The degree of oedema will increase with time, so that early intubation is imperative if there are any features of airway involvement. Laryngoscopy after an airway burn can be very difficult as surrounding oedema can make the vocal cords unrecognisable. Intubation should be undertaken by an expert, who will need to consider alternative methods such as fibre-optic bronchoscopy. Emergency cricothyroidotomy must be considered if intubation cannot be achieved by other means.

If there is *any* concern about involvement of the airway, intubation must be achieved before transfer to the burns unit. The risk for losing control of the airway en route is otherwise too high. The patient may also need to be intubated if there has been inhalation of carbon particles or toxic fumes, leading to tracheobronchitis and pneumonitis.

Intravenous access must be secure. Fluid resuscitation is at first guided by the percentage burn and patient's weight. The burn surface area is estimated using the "Rule of Nines" (Figure 12.1) or the more accurate Lund–Browder charts. Alternatively, the patient's hand (palm and fingers) is approximately 1% of the body surface area. A commonly used formula is presented in Box 12.2.

---

**Box 12.2.  Estimating fluid requirements after burns**

In the first 24 hours after a burn, **additional estimated fluid requirements = 2–4 ml** *per* **kg** *per* **percent body surface burn**.

- Remember, the time starts when the burn occurred, not when the patient arrives at hospital.
- Use physiological saline, e.g. Hartmann's solution or 0.9% saline.
- Aim to give half of this fluid in the first eight hours and the other half in the remaining 16 hours.
- Modify the fluid administered in response to the patient's observations and on the basis of advice from the receiving burns unit.

---

All such formulae are intended only as a guide to the amount of fluid required. The management should be adjusted according to the patient's response in heart rate, blood pressure, peripheral perfusion, urine output and changes in haemoglobin, sodium, and urea. Each regional burns unit may use variations on standard formulae. In communicating with the unit prior to transfer, it is important to follow specialist advice and to agree fluid management plans en route in order to provide seamless care. Until the handover at the receiving centre has been completed, the ultimate responsibility remains with the transferring team.

The patient may lose heat very quickly as a result of using cold water to stop the burning process at the scene and exposing the body surface in hospital, compounded by evaporation from the exuding burns. Children, with their high body surface area to mass ratio, are particularly prone to hypothermia. Covering the burns with clean linen or bubble wrap will help to keep the patient warm and at the same time help to control the pain. Antibiotic cream should not be applied before transfer – the receiving team will only wash it off to reassess the burns later.

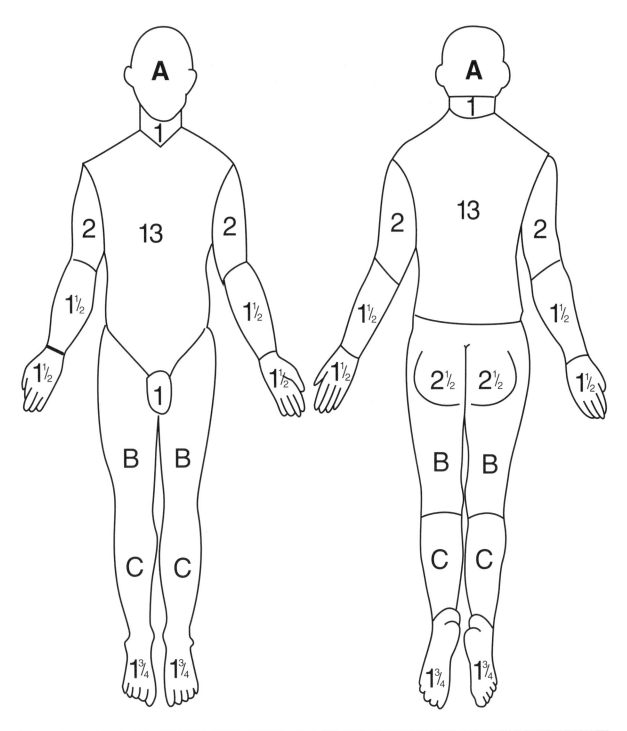

| Area | Age 0 | 1 | 5 | 10 | 15 | Adult |
|------|-------|---|---|----|----|-------|
| A = 1/2 of head | 9·5 | 8·5 | 6·5 | 5·5 | 4·5 | 3·5 |
| B = 1/2 of one thigh | 2·75 | 3·25 | 4 | 4·5 | 4·5 | 4·75 |
| C = 1/2 of one leg | 2·5 | 2·5 | 2·75 | 3·25 | 3·25 | 3·5 |

**Figure 12.1.** Body surface area (per cent). (Reproduced courtesy of Smith & Nephew Pharmaceuticals Ltd)

Partial thickness burns are more painful than full thickness burns. Pain relief should be administered as an intravenous opioid (e.g. morphine) in small increments.

Electrical burns are a particular concern as they may cause deep tissue injury even in the presence of seemingly minor entrance and exit wounds. The surface area of the burn is not a guide to the extent of the injury. The electrical current tends to be conducted along neurovascular bundles, damaging these structures and causing swelling deep within muscle compartments. Careful observation for deeper tissue injury should be maintained. Fasciotomy may be required to relieve a compartment syndrome. Myoglobinuria can result from muscle damage, leading to renal failure. In addition, electrical burns can cause cardiac arrhythmias.

In circumferential burns to the trunk or limbs, the constriction may cause respiratory embarrassment or limb ischaemia, respectively. Escharotomy is occasionally required. It is rare for this to be needed within the first six hours, so that it is more likely to be performed after transfer.

Patients with burns covering more than 20% of the body surface area may experience nausea, vomiting, and gastric distension. It is essential that these patients receive a gastric tube prior to transfer.

## Transfer of patients with spinal fractures and spinal cord injuries to a spinal unit

All patients who have sustained serious blunt trauma are suspected of having suffered a spinal injury. Spinal precautions are maintained from the outset. The whole spine should be immobilised in a neutral position on a firm, tiltable surface. The cervical spine may be controlled manually or with a combination of a hard cervical collar, side head supports, and strapping. It should be recognised that spinal immobilisation devices may interfere with the identification and management of life threatening conditions. They should be removed for examination or for specific interventions, such as intubation. Manual immobilisation should then be reinstated following such procedures.

As the examination proceeds, the spinal injury will be defined, together with any involvement of the spinal cord, from reported symptoms (pain, weakness, sensory disturbance), signs (tenderness, swelling, deformity, motor weakness, sensory impairment, abnormal breathing pattern, bradycardia, hypotension), and investigations (plain radiographs, CT scan, MRI scan).

Initial assessment of the patient with a spinal injury includes the breathing pattern, which may be compromised by paralysis of the diaphragm and intercostal muscles from a spinal cord injury. The nerve supply to the diaphragm is provided by C3–5. Complete injuries to the cord above this level are incompatible with spontaneous breathing. If the diaphragm's nerve supply is intact, the loss of the intercostals may still cause an impaired ability to take deep breaths and cough. The level of motor weakness after spinal cord injury may rise as cord oedema develops. This may put an unprotected airway at risk during transfer between hospitals.

If there is a high spinal cord injury, neurogenic shock may develop as a result of interruption of the sympathetic nerve supply to the heart and the blood vessels below the level of the cord lesion. Just as cerebral perfusion pressure must be maintained after a brain injury, so it is important to maintain sufficient blood pressure to perfuse an injured spinal cord. To this end, it is important to control haemorrhage from other injuries promptly. Generally, the blood pressure can be restored with fluid therapy, without resorting to the use of inotropes.

Patients with spinal injuries must have spinal precautions maintained, until a senior orthopaedic or specialist spinal surgeon declares that the spinal injury is stable and does not warrant their continuation. This does *not* mean that patients should remain on a spinal board for several hours. This may cause pressure sores, which will be particularly troublesome in patients with altered sensation from a spinal cord injury. The firm surface of an emergency department trolley is suitable for continuing care during stabilisation prior to transfer. For transfer itself, the spinal board may be reapplied for a short journey if no other arrangements can be made. A vacuum mattress conforming to the patient's body shape is a better solution at this stage. Provided that the ambulance trolley has a firm surface and the patient can be secured to it with firm padding to prevent sideways rocking movements en route, it is possible to transfer safely without a board. Whatever method is chosen, this should be agreed with the Ambulance Service in advance, rather than devising makeshift solutions at the time of transfer.

Patients with unstable spinal injuries may need to undergo definitive operative stabilisation before transfer, if the expertise is available locally. Of particular urgency is the patient with a partial cord injury who should also receive high dose steroids, as the current evidence suggests that this improves the outcome. There is some variation in the drugs and doses recommended, depending on local preferences, but many choose to follow Bracken's recommendations (Box 12.3).

---

**Box 12.3.   Steroid administration in spinal cord injury**

**Methyl prednisolone 30 mg kg$^{-1}$ over 1 hour**
*followed by*
**5·4 mg kg$^{-1}$ hr$^{-1}$ for the next 23 hours**

---

Tertiary hospitals serving as the major trauma unit for a geographical region should have specialist spinal surgeons on site, together with the imaging required for planning definitive care (e.g. CT and MRI scanning). Spinal injury units are supraregional facilities specialising in spinal cord rehabilitation and may not have all other surgical specialties on site. The patient must have other injuries stabilised before contemplating transfer to such isolated units.

Transporting a patient with an unstable spinal injury requires a smooth journey at a steady speed. It is not necessary to crawl along, spending unnecessary hours in transit. Of course, sudden acceleration or deceleration and rapid cornering must be avoided. A police escort is of great value in preventing other road users from interfering with the smooth passage. Transfer by helicopter is a useful alternative, avoiding bumps and potholes in the road, but if the helipads are remote from the hospital, secondary transfers by land ambulance may be required, reducing the benefits.

## Transfer of patients with other injuries

Most hospitals receiving major trauma patients have in-house specialists capable of managing most orthopaedic injuries. Nevertheless, the patient may need to be transferred out for other injuries or because no bed is available locally. An unstable pelvic injury is a life threatening emergency at risk of massive arterial or venous bleeding. Major venous bleeding is much more common and can usually be controlled by applying an external fixator to restore alignment and reduce the volume of the pelvis. External fixation should be rapidly available in all hospitals which receive major trauma patients. Major arterial bleeding is harder to control and is usually best achieved by angiography and embolisation, requiring the availability of an interventional radiologist. Definitive care of unstable pelvic or acetabular injuries may require internal fixation, which is best performed in a specialist centre. This can usually wait a few days until the patient's condition has been fully stabilised, though some traumatologists advocate early operative intervention.

Not all hospitals have maxillofacial surgeons on site. Moreover, it is rare for the facial injury to be the reason for an acute transfer. Indeed, many such injuries can be left for several days without harm, provided that open wounds are closed. Occasionally, major airway bleeding can occur, particularly in association with Le Fort type 3 fractures. Nasal packs or balloons may be required to tamponade bleeding into the nasopharynx.

Many severe liver injuries can be managed conservatively but require careful observation and the means of intervention in the event of deterioration. In high risk injuries, this may be best achieved at a regional surgical liver unit. If cardiovascular stability cannot be achieved before transfer, laparotomy must be performed and the liver packed. The surgical technique is critical, compressing the liver from outside rather than inserting swabs into a laceration or defect, which only worsens the bleeding by holding wound edges apart. At the same time, transfusion with warmed blood, fresh frozen plasma, and platelets will be required. If temporary control can be achieved, a window of opportunity presents in which rapid transfer to a liver unit is possible. Transferring such a patient with a high risk of exsanguination represents one of the most difficult of all situations requiring transfer.

## TRANSFERS FOR MEDICAL AND NON-TRAUMA SURGICAL CONDITIONS

Medical problems in adults, especially the elderly, represent a current epidemic, placing hospitals under strain and forcing transfers because of the lack of free beds. The expertise to deal with most acute medical conditions is available within the district general hospitals to which the patients present. In this sense, most medical transfers are "overflow" patients between equivalent facilities, rather than from generalists to specialists. Extending the provision of critical care beds at a local or national level is required to reduce the number of these potentially unnecessary transfers.

One reason why this problem has arisen is increasing expectation. Increasing capability of interhospital transfer itself may also be contributing to the escalating demand to transfer patients requiring active resuscitation.

Other medical or surgical patients require transfer to specialist units for investigation or intervention. Acute cardiac intervention in worsening angina and valvular or septal rupture is increasingly undertaken. The interventions may involve cardiologists (e.g. angioplasty) or cardiac surgeons (e.g. emergency coronary artery bypass grafting, valve replacement or septal repair). Similarly, neurologists and neurosurgeons are accepting more patients for acute intervention, such as clipping or coiling intracranial aneurysms.

While the reasons for transfer following trauma reflect anatomical sites of injury and the corresponding surgical specialties, medical conditions fall into physiological categories (Box 12.4). The diversity of medical conditions requires a classification that extends further than the conventional ABCD of the various advanced life support courses. By expanding beyond the respiratory, circulatory and nervous systems to include metabolism/excretion and host defence, the vast majority of medical conditions can be incorporated conveniently. Metabolism/excretion refers to biochemical processes and includes renal, hepatic, gastro-intestinal and endocrine problems. Host defence represents the interaction between the body as a whole and external influences. As such, it encompasses infection, immunity, inflammation and intoxication (from foreign substances).

Medical conditions sometimes affect a single system, but it is multi-system failure that challenges the transferring team the most. The prognosis worsens as more systems fail and the impact of each system on every other system becomes apparent.

## Box 12.4. Medical conditions requiring transfer

**Respiration (AB)**

Respiratory failure (to a respiratory physician, intensivist or *rarely* to an extracorporeal membrane oxygenation (ECMO) unit)
- Acute severe asthma, chronic obstructive airways disease
- Severe pneumonia
- Adult respiratory distress syndrome (ARDS)

**Circulation (C)**

Critical ischaemic heart disease (to a cardiologist or cardiac surgeon)
- Unstable angina, myocardial infarction
- Heart failure, cardiogenic shock
- Arrhythmia
- Valvular or septal rupture

Other cardiac disease (to a cardiologist)
- Cardiomyopathy, myocarditis, pericarditis

Critical vascular insufficiency (to a vascular surgeon)
- Aortic aneurysm or dissection
- Limb ischaemia

**Nervous system (D)**

Central nervous system failure (to a neurologist, neurosurgeon, spinal surgeon, stroke unit or psychiatric unit)
- Intracerebral haemorrhage or infarction
- Intracranial abscess, encephalitis or meningitis
- Intracranial tumour or hydrocephalus
- Spinal cord compression
- Acute psychosis or suicidal behaviour

Peripheral nervous system failure (to a neurologist)
- Myasthenia gravis
- Guillain–Barré syndrome (postinfectious polyneuropathy)

**Metabolism/excretion**

Metabolic failure (to a renal, hepatic, gastrointestinal or endocrine unit)
- Renal failure
- Acute liver failure
- Variceal or other gastrointestinal haemorrhage
- Diabetic ketoacidosis or lactic acidosis
- Thyrotoxicosis or other endocrine/metabolic derangement

**Host defence**

Infection (to an infectious diseases unit or ICU)
- Septic shock including meningococcaemia
- Specific infections

Immune failure (to a specialist immunological unit, haematologist or oncologist)
- Severe allergy or autoimmune process
- Immune deficiency or marrow suppression

Intoxication (to an ICU or specific poisons unit, e.g. hyperbaric unit)
- Poisoning/overdose
- Carbon monoxide poisoning

Immersion/other environmental injury (to an ICU)
- Near drowning
- Hypothermia

## Respiratory failure

Patients requiring transfer with respiratory failure will generally require intubation and ventilation. In acute severe asthma, chronic obstructive airways disease (COAD), severe pneumonia or adult respiratory distress syndrome (ARDS), there may be particular difficulties in ventilation. The airway pressures may be high and the portable ventilator must be capable of providing satisfactory ventilation. PEEP may be needed, especially in ARDS and in severe pneumonia. The ventilator may have an in-built facility to provide PEEP or a manual PEEP valve can be added to the circuit.

While most cases can be managed adequately with the standard inspired to expired time ratio (I:E ratio) of 1:2, the ability to modify inspiratory and expiratory times is valuable in complex cases. ARDS, in particular, is often best managed with an inverse I:E ratio, i.e. inspiratory time greater than the expiratory time. On the other hand, bronchospasm may require prolonged expiratory times to allow the lungs to empty adequately.

## Circulatory failure

Ischaemic heart disease is the commonest threat to life in older people. Cardiologists and cardiac surgeons offer the possibility of revascularisation by angioplasty or coronary artery grafting, respectively. Transporting a patient with critically unstable angina or acute myocardial infarction is a hazardous procedure, with attendant risks of arrhythmia, heart failure, and cardiogenic shock.

After myocardial infarction, intravenous analgesia and thrombolytic therapy (unless contraindicated) should be administered without delay. If a patient with a proven diagnosis of myocardial infarction is in an area where thrombolytic drugs are not available or where it is considered unsafe for their administration, transfer to the coronary care unit (CCU) should be arranged as a *critical* case, even if the patient's vital signs are normal. If streptokinase (or an equivalent drug) has been administered in the emergency department, then it may be wise to keep the patient under observation in the high dependency environment of the resuscitation room for up to one hour. The patient can then be transferred to the CCU as an *ill and unstable* case.

Rhythm disorders should be controlled whenever possible before transfer, using cardioversion or antiarrhythmic drugs as indicated. The transferring team must be proficient in CPR and be able to defibrillate or institute alternative antiarrhythmic therapy en route in an emergency.

Heart failure is a gratifying condition to treat, usually responding well to diuretics and vasodilators. Intubation and inotropes are rarely needed. Cardiogenic shock, on the other hand, has a very high mortality. If available, an intra-aortic balloon pump (IABP) may be inserted via the femoral artery. By alternately inflating in diastole to maintain coronary perfusion and deflating during systole to reduce afterload, the cardiac output may be much improved. Patients may be transferred with an IABP *in situ*, as most are equipped with a satisfactory battery. The machines themselves tend to be bulky and provide logistic challenges to escorts. The IABP should be regarded as a specialist tool and an experienced cardiologist, cardiac surgeon or specialist technician should accompany the patient during transfer.

An increasingly common transfer between hospitals is for patients who have had a cardiac arrest from which they have been successfully resuscitated in terms of their heart, but who have not fully regained consciousness. These patients require intensive care, provided that their overall prognosis is not so poor as to render such care futile. The fact that such transfers are a regular occurrence reflects the lack of available intensive care beds.

Critical peripheral vascular disease is not infrequent in a population with a high prevalence of atherosclerosis. Leaking aortic aneurysms are best operated on immediately at the hospital where they present, provided that a capable surgeon is available. As not all hospitals have specialist vascular surgeons on site, this poses a risk–benefit conundrum. Do we subject the patient to immediate surgery in less capable hands or risk the patient dying en route to the specialist vascular surgeon? Alternative arrangements are feasible depending on local circumstances. For example, the local surgeon may be able to control the bleeding immediately, while the vascular surgeon travels from another hospital to join in the operation later. Such a solution is inevitably a compromise as it depletes the other hospital of a surgeon and is only feasible if adequate cover can be provided.

## Nervous system failure

In terms of transfer, life threatening intracranial problems are generally managed in a similar way to head injuries. Maintaining perfusion pressure and reducing intracranial pressure are of similar concern. In intracranial infections (meningitis, encephalitis, abscess), high dose antibiotics are indicated and should be started as soon as possible, immediately after taking blood for culture. For suspected bacterial infections, drugs which cover likely organisms and penetrate well into the brain, such as ceftriaxone, are preferred. For suspected viral encephalitis, acyclovir is administered.

Subarachnoid haemorrhage should be managed according to the severity of the bleed, as indicated by the patient's clinical state and appearance on the CT scan. High blood pressure may precipitate a further bleed, which may be catastrophic. Preventing surges of blood pressure by gentle handling, good analgesia, judicious sedation and, if intubation is required, by well judged anaesthetic agent doses is very important. At the same time, vasospasm is a risk in this condition and local brain perfusion may be compromised by low blood pressure. Nimodipine is used to reduce vasospasm, but may itself cause hypotension.

In general, spinal cord compression from non-traumatic causes is managed in a similar way to spinal cord injuries. There may be less risk of further damage en route compared with an unstable fracture, but gentle handling and maintenance of blood pressure remain cornerstones of practice.

Peripheral nervous system failure, as in myasthenia gravis and Guillain–Barré syndrome, may cause sufficient weakness to precipitate respiratory failure, which is compounded by an ineffective cough. Such patients are often sicker than they appear and it is essential that the transferring team recognises any deterioration requiring intubation and ventilation. These patients do not necessarily show the usual signs of respiratory distress. Their weakness prevents them from revealing the furrowed brow, intercostal or sternal recession or the prominent use of accessory muscles.

## Metabolic failure

Where renal dialysis or haemofiltration is not available, patients with severe oliguric renal failure need to be transferred. Most intensive care units can provide haemofiltration in house and assume responsibility for cases of acute renal failure, consulting with renal specialists when indicated. Nevertheless, some cases will need to be transferred. Once fluid overload, acidosis, and life threatening hyperkalaemia have been controlled by haemofiltration or haemodialysis, transfer becomes a much safer possibility. Without these forms of treatment, serious hyperkalaemia must be controlled temporarily by treatments such as insulin and glucose to help prevent cardiac compromise en route. Attention to detail is needed to achieve appropriate fluid balance in these patients. If they are anuric or severely oliguric, it is easy to accidentally overload them with fluid. If they are in a diuretic phase of renal failure, failure to keep pace with the urinary loss can lead to hypovolaemia and serious electrolyte imbalance.

Diabetes insipidus is a metabolic disorder in which excessive losses can occur, elevating the sodium concentration and causing serious dehydration within a few hours. In this situation, stopping the diuresis with desmopressin (DDAVP) is the appropriate management, rather than just replacing losses.

Diabetic ketoacidosis also leads to fluid depletion and acidosis. In this case, it is important to replace losses intravenously and to administer insulin by infusion. At the same time, the cause of the episode should be considered, e.g. a precipitating infection. These patients should not be transferred until they are stable, with the dehydration, acidosis, and hyperglycaemia well controlled. In these circumstances, complete fluid replacement takes place over 24 hours or longer, rather than over a few hours, to avoid osmotic shifts which can lead to cerebral oedema. Waiting this long to transfer is not necessary, but the patient should at least undergo initial treatment to restore the central venous pressure and peripheral perfusion, to reduce the blood glucose to less than $20 \, \text{mmol} \, l^{-1}$ and to improve the pH to over 7·3.

Hepatic and gastrointestinal disorders may be associated with life threatening haemorrhage, but are considered in the *metabolic* rather than *circulatory* category as they are generally managed by clinicians whose main focus is within the metabolic domain. In liver failure, bleeding may result from clotting disorders or from oesophageal varices. Treatment with fresh frozen plasma, vitamin K and, occasionally, a Sengstaken tube may be indicated to control bleeding before transfer. Liver failure may give rise to acute confusional states or coma and the patients are also prone to develop renal failure.

## Host defence failure

Severe infections should be managed with targeted antibiotics before transfer. If laboratory evidence is available, the choice will depend on confirmed or projected organism sensitivities. Otherwise, specimens are sent, microbiological advice is taken and a best guess is made. Septicaemia in its severe form is a multisystem disorder causing *respiratory* failure from shunting or ARDS, *circulatory* failure from myocardial depression, systemic vasodilation and disseminated intravascular coagulation, *nervous system* failure from a toxic confusional state, *metabolic* failure from renal impairment and other *host defence* failure from bone marrow suppression. In addition, immune processes may play a part in the pathophysiology of the disease itself, e.g. the petechial haemorrhages in meningococcal septicaemia. Achieving stability prior to transfer is a key goal in these cases.

Poisoning does not generally necessitate transfer between hospitals. Most cases can be managed locally, with advice from a regional or national poisons centre. However, these patients still provide a challenge to transfer safely within the hospital, from the emergency department or medical admissions unit to the ICU or high dependency ward. Patients with tricyclic antidepressant overdose can be particularly unstable, suffering intractable arrhythmias, seizures, and coma.

Carbon monoxide poisoning may be intentional from a suicide attempt or accidental from a faulty domestic heating appliance. Severe cases require transfer to a supraregional hyperbaric unit to reduce secondary brain injury. Carbon monoxide has a much higher affinity for haemoglobin than does oxygen, impeding oxygen delivery to the tissues. It is essential to transfer rapidly and to maintain ventilation with 100% oxygen en route.

## PAEDIATRIC TRANSFERS

Children pose particular problems because of their range of shapes and sizes and their different physiological and psychological behaviour. They suffer from many of the same conditions as adults and are prone to their own specific problems. Sick children generate anxiety in their carers, not all of whom are familiar or confident with paediatric intensive care methods.

Sick or injured children may initially be taken to a hospital capable of carrying out resuscitation and stabilisation, but unable to offer definitive care. The children will need to be transported elsewhere. Critically ill children transferred by untrained personnel have been shown to suffer transfer related morbidity which is largely preventable. In the United Kingdom, a standard of practice for the transport of critically ill children has been set by the Paediatric Intensive Care Society. As non-specialists have become more aware of the risks of transfer, specialised paediatric retrieval teams based at paediatric intensive care units are increasingly called upon to transfer sick children.

Some transfers are inherently time-critical, e.g. an expanding extradural haematoma with a dilating pupil. In such cases, the time taken to mobilise the specialist retrieval team and for them to travel to the referring hospital and take over care may prejudice the outcome. Helicopters may be used to speed up the "time to specialist take-over", provided that the helicopter itself can be mobilised rapidly and dispatched to pick up the retrieval team. Otherwise, these time-critical transfers are by necessity carried out by the referring team, in liaison with the receiving unit. In order for this to be an effective long term solution, the specialist unit must take responsibility in providing an educational outreach service to help maintain skills and knowledge in the surrounding hospitals.

In contrast to the time-critical transfers for life saving surgery at the receiving hospital, most critically ill children need continuing resuscitation and stabilisation rather than immediate transfer. It may take a retrieval team several hours or indeed all day to achieve sufficient stability for safe transfer. Severe meningococcal septicaemia often falls into this category. The vehicle which takes the retrieval team to the referring hospital cannot be expected to wait indefinitely and may be redeployed until required. When rebooking a suitable land or air ambulance for the *intensive* transfer back, the 20-minute guideline (see Figure 5.1) allows the team to collect together equipment and recheck blood gas values before the ambulance arrives.

The referring department should embark on joint management as early as possible with the clinicians who will be transporting the patient. This applies whether the team is from the same hospital or is a specialist retrieval team from the receiving unit. Overall responsibility lies initially with the referring clinicians and should be provided at senior level. When it shifts to the receiving unit will depend on the type of transfer. In a retrieval, the team from the receiving hospital will assume overall responsibility at the referring hospital at an agreed time after a handover period. If the transfer is carried out by the referring unit, the responsibility is maintained throughout transportation and continued until the handover at the destination has been completed.

Even in urgent situations, it is essential to evaluate, resuscitate, and attempt to stabilise the child before setting off. Whatever the injury or illness, the airway must be secure and the ventilation must be adequate. Intravenous access must be established and life saving drugs and fluids administered. A thorough examination should be performed to exclude the need to carry out other emergency procedures prior to transportation. Baseline haematological and biochemical samples should have been taken when the intravenous lines were placed and essential imaging carried out.

Dedicated transport equipment for monitoring and treatment should be available in the emergency department. Familiarity with such equipment is a prerequisite for all emergency staff involved in the transport of critically ill children. A list of essential equipment is shown in Box 12.5.

---

**Box 12.5.  Paediatric transfer equipment**

**Airway**

1. Oropharyngeal airway sizes 000, 00, 0, 1, 2, 3
2. Endotracheal tubes sizes 2·5–7·5 mm uncuffed (in 0·5 mm steps) and 7·5 cuffed
3. Laryngoscopes:

   - straight paediatric blades
   - adult curved blade

4. Magill forceps
5. Yankauer sucker, portable powered suction device (manual or battery) and endobronchial suction tubes
6. Needle cricothyroidotomy set

**Breathing**

1. Oxygen masks (with reservoir bag)
2. Self-inflating bags (with reservoir bag):

   - 500 ml child size
   - 1600 ml adult size

3. Face masks:

   - infant – circular 01, 1, 2
   - child – anatomical 2, 3
   - adult – anatomical 4, 5

4. Connectors and catheter mounts
5. T-piece and open-ended bag
6. Infant and child portable ventilator
7. Capnograph
8. Chest drain set

**Circulation**

1. ECG monitor – defibrillator (with paediatric paddles)
2. Blood pressure monitor – invasive and non-invasive (with infant and child-sized cuffs)
3. Pulse oximeter (with infant and child-sized probes)
4. Intravenous access requirements:

   - intravenous cannulae (as available) 18–25 G
   - intraosseous infusion needles 16–18 G
   - paediatric central venous lines
   - graduated burette
   - intravenous giving sets
   - syringes 1–50 ml
   - syringe pumps

5. Intravenous drip monitoring device
6. Cutdown set

**Fluids**

1. 0·9% saline
2. Hartmann's solution or Ringer's lactate
3. 4% dextrose and 0·18% saline
4. 5% and 10% dextrose
5. Colloid (including human albumin solution)

**Drugs**

1. Epinephrinenaline 1:10 000 and 1:1000
2. Atropine 0·6 or 1 mg/ml
3. Sodium bicarbonate 8·4% (more dilute for infants)
4. Lignocaine 1%, amiodarone
5. Dextrose 10% and 50%
6. Calcium chloride 10%
7. Frusemide 20 mg/ml
8. Mannitol 10% or 20%
9. Other inotropes (e.g. dopamine, norepinephrine)
10. Antibiotics (penicillin, gentamicin, amoxicillin, flucloxacillin, cefotaxime)

**Miscellaneous**

1. Stick test for glucose
2. Paediatric resuscitation chart or tape
3. Paediatric spine board
4. Infant incubator
5. Nasogastric tubes
6. Chemical warming packs (for infants)
7. Scissors, tape

---

It is often stressed that children are different from adults. While this is a vital consideration, children suffer from many of the same conditions as adults and the overall approach to their care is similar. Box 12.6 lists the reasons for transferring children, mirroring the indications discussed for adults but pointing out important differences.

**Box 12.6. Paediatric conditions requiring transfer**

| | |
|---|---|
| **Trauma** | As adults, taking into account differences, **plus** |

- Non-accidental injury
- Growth plate (Salter-type) orthopaedic injuries

**Non-trauma Respiration (AB)**    Respiratory failure

- Acute severe asthma
- Severe pneumonia
- Bronchiolitis
- Cystic fibrosis
- Bronchopulmonary dysplasia
- Croup, epiglottitis
- Inhaled foreign body

**Circulation (C)**    Congenital heart disease (to a paediatric cardiologist or cardiac surgeon)

- Structural abnormalities
- Heart failure, cyanotic episodes, arrhythmia

Other heart disease (to a paediatric cardiologist or PICU)
- Myocarditis, pericarditis

**Nervous system (D)**    Central nervous system failure (to a paediatric neurologist, neurosurgeon or PICU)

- Intracranial abscess, encephalitis or meningitis
- Intracranial tumour or hydrocephalus
- Cerebral palsy

**Metabolism/excretion**    Metabolic failure (to a specialist paediatric unit)

- Renal failure
- Acute liver failure
- Hyper- and hypoglycaemia
- Other congenital/acquired endocrine/metabolic derangement

**Host defence**    Infection (to an infectious diseases unit or PICU)

- Septic shock including meningococcaemia
- Specific infections

Immune failure (to a specialist immunological unit, haematologist or oncologist)

- Severe allergy or autoimmune process
- Immune deficiency or marrow suppression

Intoxication (to an ICU or specific poisons unit, e.g. hyperbaric unit)

- Poisoning/overdose
- Carbon monoxide poisoning

Immersion

- Near drowning
- Hypothermia

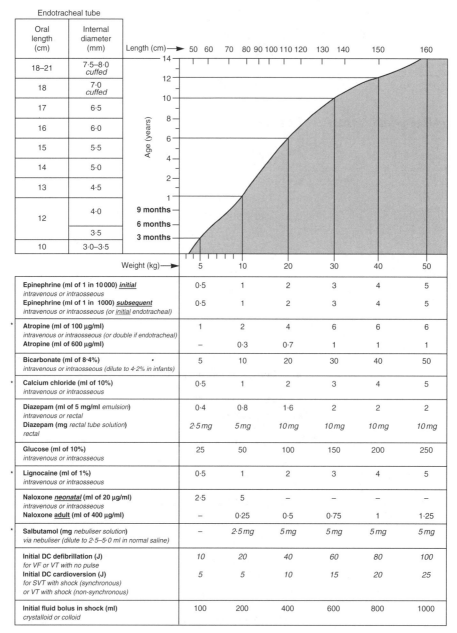

**Figure 12.2.** Paediatric resuscitation chart.

# Trauma

Trauma is the commonest cause of death and a potent cause of long term disability in children over the age of one year. As in adults, head injury accounts for most of the deaths and is the commonest injury requiring interhospital transfer. Trauma is managed in children with the same priorities as in adults and according to the same general principles. The nature of the injuries sustained varies according to anatomical differences. For example, their pliable ribs require more force to fracture and their immature long bones have growth plates, which are vulnerable to particular fracture patterns as described in the Salter classification. As pedestrians, they are shorter in stature and are struck by road vehicles at a different level on the body, transmitting forces to different structures. Children are less likely to be involved in serious interpersonal violence, although non-accidental injury must always be considered in infants and young children with multiple injuries.

Children's emotional needs are different, especially when they are sick, and they need continuing education and play as they recover. For these reasons alone, they need to be transferred to a specific paediatric environment. In terms of their medical management, injuries needing operative care in an adult can often be managed conservatively. Clinical governance requires their care to be carried out by clinicians who specialise in children's injuries and manage sufficient cases per year to maintain their expertise.

Children have immature nervous systems, which makes them vulnerable to misjudgements leading to injury and also makes them harder to assess – if you cannot yet talk, you cannot explain what the problem is or how it happened. They are highly dependent on their parents and become anxious in their absence. These factors make children who remain awake during transfer a challenge to care for. Those with more critical injuries who are sedated, intubated and ventilated are of even more concern, even to experienced clinicians. "Controlled paranoia", however, is a healthy attitude in escorts, who must watch constantly for signs of deterioration and for evidence of missed injuries.

## Non-trauma

### Respiratory failure

Children are prone to respiratory infections. Their upper and lower airways are smaller and more easily obstructed by mucosal swelling, secretions or a foreign body. They may desaturate frighteningly quickly. In infancy, the respiratory muscles are relatively underdeveloped and inefficient. The small size of the trachea makes it all too easy for the endotracheal tube to become dislodged during transfer, making secure fixation of paramount importance. It is also important to be aware that flexion and extension of the neck tend to move the tube downwards or upwards, respectively.

Endotracheal tubes should be uncuffed in children up to puberty. The tube sizes are estimated from the formula:

$$\text{Endotracheal tube size (internal diameter in mm)} = [\text{age in years}/4] + 4$$

The alternative rule of thumb is the size of the child's little finger or the size that will just snugly fit into the nostril. Ventilation rate is higher in small children, reflecting their increased metabolic rate and oxygen consumption. Transport ventilators suitable for adults can often be used in children down to the age of 12 months. Infants, on the other hand, have different needs. Pressure controlled systems are preferable to compensate for leaks and to protect against inadvertent barotrauma. PEEP is generally regarded as essential when ventilating small children.

Upper airway obstruction associated with acute epiglottitis is now thankfully rare in the UK, owing to immunisation against haemophilus B infection. Intubation by an expert in anaesthesia and careful tube fixation are essential before transfer between hospitals in this condition. Viral laryngotracheobronchitis or croup also causes upper airway obstruction and is generally a mild, self-limiting condition. It remains important to recognise fulminating cases which need intubation and to remember that as the condition affects the airway at different levels, the trachea will be narrowed and a smaller than usual endotracheal tube size needed.

Bronchiolitis is a specific condition of infancy mainly but not always associated with respiratory syncytial virus infection (RSV). Ex-premature babies and those with chronic lung or congenital heart conditions are prone to the serious complications of bronchiolitis, such as exhaustion, apnoea, respiratory failure, and heart failure.

*Circulatory failure*

Cardiac arrest and life threatening arrhythmias are rare in childhood. Nevertheless, the transfer team must be proficient in their management. As with respiratory deterioration, a child's circulatory state can worsen precipitously. Vascular access is often more difficult, especially in the chubby infant or toddler. Although at least two intravenous lines should be in place before setting off on a transfer, intraosseous cannulation must be available en route. For hypovolaemia, fluid boluses should be administered. The standard aliquot of fluid is 20 ml kg$^{-1}$ and is best worked out in a small child by using a 20 ml syringe and giving the same number of syringe-fulls as the child's estimated body weight in kilograms.

Congenital heart disease comprises a complex set of conditions which baffle the non-expert. Simple ABCD principles still apply, but there are unique problems. In some malformations, the child's survival is dependent on patency of the ductus arteriosus, which connects the aorta and pulmonary trunk. Prostaglandin infusions may be needed to help keep it patent until corrective surgery can take place. Congenital heart problems by their very nature tend to present within a few days of birth and the infant may need to be transferred to a supraregional paediatric cardiac unit at this vulnerable time. In severe cases, specialist retrieval teams should be used, as few general clinicians have the necessary training and experience to manage these cases well.

Children rarely suffer from heart failure in the absence of congenital heart disease, though it can occur as a complication of viral myocarditis in previously well children. The management involves giving oxygen, careful fluid balance and treatment with diuretics, digoxin, vasodilators, and inotropes, usually in liaison with the supraregional paediatric cardiac centre.

In monitoring heart failure in children, observations are made of colour, capillary return, pulse rate and rhythm, blood pressure, central venous pressure, and urinary output. In infants, liver distension is a useful additional sign of heart failure.

*Nervous system failure*

Children are prone to fits, particularly in the face of an escalating fever. Children with developmental neurological disorders may have intractable seizures, which do not respond to conventional drug therapy. Seizures may also reflect a serious underlying pathological process, such as meningitis. It is wise to suspect such an intracranial infection in fitting or comatose children with no obvious alternative diagnosis and treat them vigorously with antibiotics. It is imperative not to forget to measure the blood glucose in these children to exclude hypoglycaemia. Hypo- and hypernatremia are other treatable causes of convulsions.

Children with fits usually respond well to benzodiazepines administered rectally or intravenously and will rarely need transfer as an emergency. Occasionally, fitting may persist despite a combination of anticonvulsants. If alternative drugs, such as paraldehyde and phenytoin, are ineffective, a barbiturate infusion may be required. In this situation, the child will need to be intubated and ventilated in anticipation of the respiratory depression that will accompany high dose barbiturates, especially in combination with other sedative anticonvulsants. Though muscle relaxants must be used to facilitate intubation, it is then sensible to avoid them so that the occurrence of fits may be noted clinically. At the same time as stabilising the child, a careful search must be made for the underlying cause. If the cause is uncertain, an urgent CT should be performed to exclude surgically treatable causes, such as a cerebral abscess or hydrocephalus. The child will need to be transferred to a paediatric intensive care unit.

*Metabolic failure*

Metabolic disorders such as diabetes ketoacidosis and acute renal failure are managed along the same general lines as in adults. Inborn errors of metabolism are specific to childhood, as is Reye's syndrome, which is characterised by hypoglycaemia, altered consciousness, and hepatomegaly with liver dysfunction. Young children are especially vulnerable to hypoglycaemia, as are adolescents who have drunk excessive alcohol.

Young children are less able to concentrate their urine and so need to pass more for their size to eliminate the waste products. Passing $1\,\text{ml}\,\text{kg}^{-1}\,\text{hr}^{-1}$ in larger children or $2\,\text{ml}\,\text{kg}^{-1}\,\text{hr}^{-1}$ in infants is regarded as adequate. In small boys, passing a urinary catheter is associated with a risk of subsequent urethral stricture. A catheter should only be inserted if there is a good indication and the procedure should be performed gently with a well lubricated catheter (or feeding tube) of the correct size.

Frightened, anxious children tend to swallow air and sick children may suffer from gastric stasis. For these reasons, it is sometimes appropriate to insert a nasogastric tube in an awake child. In the unconscious child, it is routine practice to decompress the stomach to minimise the risk of gastric aspiration, remembering that there is no endotracheal tube cuff to help seal the airway.

*Host defence failure*

Just as fits and coma are suspected of being due to central nervous system infection (or hypoglycaemia) until proven otherwise, so a lethargic or generally ill-looking child is regarded as having underlying sepsis. The child is examined for supportive evidence of sepsis, samples are taken for microscopy and culture and, if in any doubt, antibiotics are administered.

Meningococcal disease may present as meningitis, septicaemia with cardiovascular collapse or, more rarely, as a combination. Meningococcal septicaemia has a peak incidence in childhood and is the most fulminant infectious disease. The interval from the first symptom or sign to death can be less than 12 hours. It is usually suspected on the basis of a petechial or purpuric rash in an ill-looking child, in conjunction with the history of a flu-like illness, but the rash may be absent in up to 20% of cases at presentation. Initial treatment is extremely urgent in an ill child and typically consists of the sequence of steps in Box 12.7.

A critical step in the initial management is to secure intravenous access and administer $20\,\text{ml}\,\text{kg}^{-1}$ of a colloid, such as human albumin solution (HAS). Physiological saline (0·9% saline or Hartmann's solution) is considered by some to be a suitable alternative to colloid, as there have been recent concerns over the use of HAS. These children may require several further fluid boluses to restore tissue perfusion, but in fulminant cases, they are also easily tipped over into pulmonary oedema. Antibiotics should be given without delay by the first doctor making the diagnosis.

---

**Box 12.7. Typical steps in the immediate management of suspected meningococcal septicaemia**

1. Summoning help from experts in paediatric intensive care (or if not available locally, senior paediatricians, intensivists, anaesthetists or emergency physicians)
2. Checking ABCD and intervening immediately if airway or breathing compromised
3. Administering oxygen by face mask (if A and B are OK at this stage)
4. Vascular access, by the intraosseous route if necessary
5. Fluid resuscitation with 1–2, or more, aliquots of $20\,\text{ml}\,\text{kg}^{-1}$
6. Intravenous antibiotics, e.g. high dose ceftriaxone or cefotaxime, after taking blood cultures
7. Reviewing ABCD
   - Consider intubation and ventilation if oxygenation worsening, circulation not improving or becoming more obtunded

- Proceed to central venous access and consider inotropic support, using the peripheral route initially, if a central line is not yet in place
  - Make sure hypoglycaemia has been excluded if the child is obtunded
8. Placement of other tubes and lines, e.g. arterial line, gastric tube, and urinary catheter
9. Chest radiograph to confirm tube positions
10. Continuing review of arterial blood gas results, full blood count, clotting, urea and electrolytes and glucose, together with trends in oxygen saturation, pulse rate, blood pressure, and urine output
11. Transferring to a paediatric intensive care unit

As discussed above, this process may take many hours before the team is ready to transfer. The delay in arriving in the definitive PICU is more than offset by the achievement of stability prior to transfer, provided that experienced personnel are involved and that the appropriate drugs and equipment are available.

## TRANSFERRING THE SEVERELY HEAD INJURED PATIENT: AN EXAMPLE OF ACCEPT IN PRACTICE

There are so many conditions requiring transfer, each with its own problems, that it has not been feasible to describe the care of each using the full ACCEPT system. Having outlined some aspects of care across a range of conditions in the previous sections, the full ACCEPT approach is now applied in more detail to an important specific condition – head injury.

### Assessment and control

The patient with a severe head injury is extremely susceptible to hypoxia ($PaO_2 < 60$ mmHg [8 kPa]) and hypotension (systolic blood pressure $< 90$ mmHg) (Table 12.1). Consequently, even though the patient may appear to have a patent airway and adequate ventilation, intubation and ventilation are required when there is:

- inadequate gas exchange: $PaO_2 < 67 \cdot 5$ mmHg (9 kPa) in air, $< 97 \cdot 5$ mmHg (13 kPa) on $O_2$, $PaCO_2 > 45$ mmHg (6 kPa)
- inability to protect their airway
- irregular or abnormal respiration, particularly if spontaneous hyperventilation to $PaCO_2 < 26 \cdot 25$ mmHg (3·5 kPa)
- coma, GCS $\leqslant 8$
- neurological deterioration.

**Table 12.1.** Effect of hypoxia and hypotension on outcome after transfer to neurosurgical units in USA (from the Traumatic Coma Data Bank).

| Secondary insult | Number of patients | Percentage | Outcome (%) | | |
|---|---|---|---|---|---|
| | | | Good or moderate | Severely disabled or vegetative | Dead |
| None | 456 | 65 | 51 | 22 | 27 |
| Hypoxia | 78 | 11 | 45 | 22 | 33 |
| Hypotension | 113 | 16 | 26 | 14 | 60 |
| Both | 52 | 8 | 6 | 19 | 75 |

Tracheal intubation should be facilitated by the administration of intravenous anaesthetic agents and muscle relaxants to prevent a rise in intracranial pressure (ICP). At the same time, it is important not to cause hypotension by the use of these drugs, as this can be even more harmful in reducing cerebral perfusion pressure (Box 12.8). An obtunded or shocked patient needs less anaesthetic agent to achieve the same depth of anaesthesia. It goes without saying that the person performing this task must have adequate training in the technique of intubation and sufficient anaesthetic experience to be able to judge the doses appropriately. Ventilation is best checked manually immediately after intubation before proceeding to mechanical ventilation. For continuing care, a mechanical ventilator is more consistent and should be adjusted according to the result of repeated arterial blood gas analysis.

---

**Box 12.8.  Cerebral perfusion pressure**

Cerebral perfusion pressure = mean arterial pressure − intracranial pressure
    (CPP)                              (MAP)                              (ICP)

---

The $PaO_2$ should be maintained over 97·5 mmHg (13 kPa). While a high concentration of oxygen can be harmful in the longer term, it is wise to permit a higher $PaO_2$ for transfer, giving a greater margin of safety. In patients without serious chest injuries, the $PaO_2$ will often exceed the target of 13 kPa, simply as a result of the restricted choice for the inspired oxygen setting on many transport ventilators (typically 60% or 100% oxygen).

The aim should be to ventilate the patient to achieve a $PaCO_2$ of 30–33·75 mmHg (4–4·5 kPa). Hyperventilation to a lower $PaCO_2$ is no longer recommended, as the cerebral vasoconstriction this induces may further compromise an already reduced cerebral blood flow (CBF). It should only be used in those patients who either have evidence of cerebral hyperaemia or who exhibit signs of uncal herniation during transfer, e.g. dilating pupils, extensor posturing, and Cushing's reflex.

The end-tidal carbon dioxide ($ETCO_2$) should be monitored in all intubated, ventilated head injured patients. However, it is important not to regard the $ETCO_2$ value as an accurate reflection of the $PaCO_2$ in a critically injured patient. In such circumstances, the $ETCO_2$ underestimates the $PaCO_2$, particularly if the patient is shocked. This is due to increased physiological dead space in the lungs caused by poor perfusion of upper (less dependent) parts of the lungs. The expired gas from these areas has a lower $CO_2$ concentration than those areas that equilibrate well with blood flowing through the lungs. As a result, when the $ETCO_2$ is low, it remains uncertain whether the $PaCO_2$ is also low. There is no substitute for checking an arterial blood gas sample. On the other hand, if the $ETCO_2$ is higher than 33·75 mmHg (4·5), then it is clear that the ventilation needs to be increased. Correlating the $PaCO_2$ and the $ETCO_2$ before setting off on the journey is helpful in maintaining control en route, but great care must be taken in interpreting changes in the $ETCO_2$ if there are concomitant changes in the circulatory status.

Hypotension from whatever cause must be identified and corrected, even if this means surgical intervention. A systolic BP < 95 mmHg is associated with increased mortality as a result of its reduction in cerebral perfusion pressure (CPP). Non-invasive devices are unreliable during transportation and may not detect shortlived changes. Early direct measurement of BP is essential.

In the unconscious head injured patient with possible intra-abdominal bleeding, abdominal ultrasound, abdominal CT scanning or diagnostic peritoneal lavage (DPL) should be performed in association with a CT scan of the head. Abdominal injuries needing laparotomy are more common than head injuries requiring craniotomy. Patients needing both are fortunately very rare (< 0·5%).

It is important that following the initial resuscitation, the patient's GCS is reassessed at regular intervals. Best eye opening (E), motor response (M), and verbal response (V) should all be recorded. While the single figure total for the GCS is helpful in tracking progress, a description of each response (e.g. E: eye opening to pain, M: withdrawing to pain, V: incomprehensible sounds) is more reliable and is not dependent on mental arithmetic! The GCS itself can be calculated from the descriptions at leisure. Remember, too, that the eyes may be closed by swelling, the patient may be paralysed with muscle relaxant drugs and the trachea may be intubated, affecting the EMV descriptions and precluding a meaningful score out of 15. In addition to the GCS, the presence of any lateralising signs should be noted along with the reaction of the pupils to light.

Fits cause a massive increase in cerebral metabolic activity and also interfere with respiratory function. They must be controlled promptly. Hypoglycaemia should also be remembered as a cause of fitting and treated in its own right as the brain is highly dependent on glucose as a substrate. A high index of suspicion should be maintained in infants, adolescents who have been drinking alcohol and in known diabetics, but it should be excluded in all unconscious patients. Hyperglycaemia, like hyperthermia, increases cerebral metabolic rate and should be controlled actively.

## Communication and evaluation

In a non-neurosurgical hospital, the possibility of transfer should be considered as soon as a severe head injury is suspected. Communication with a neurosurgeon takes place when sufficient information is available on which to base the decision to transfer the patient. Commonly, this takes place as soon as CT images are available. Box 12.9 shows the *minimum* amount of information required by the receiving team. Most neurosurgical units can receive the CT scan images via a telephone link, allowing an informed evaluation of the potential benefits of transfer (including operative decompression) compared with the risks. During subsequent preparation and transfer, the neurosurgeon will need to be informed of any significant change in the patient's condition, particularly if there is any neurological deterioration. In order to "buy time" the neurosurgeon may advise the administration of mannitol ($0\cdot3$–$1\,g\,kg^{-1}$) in an attempt to decrease ICP to maintain CPP.

---

**Box 12.9.   Patient details required for referral with a severe head injury**

1. Patient's age, sex, mechanism of injury, time of injury
2. Initial management

   - Airway – protected or intubated
   - Breathing – spontaneous or controlled ventilation, $PaO_2$, $PaCO_2$
   - Circulation – blood pressure, pulse rate, fluids administered, blood loss
   - Treatment of associated injuries

3. Neurological status

   - Initial neurological status; talked or not after injury
   - Status on arrival at hospital (GCS)
   - Trend since arrival and in response to resuscitation
   - Localising signs and pupillary responses
   - Fits
   - Skull fracture

---

4.  Other injuries

    - Face and neck (including cervical spine)
    - Trunk – chest, abdomen, retroperitoneum, thoracolumbar spine
    - Skin and bone – pelvis, long bones, soft tissues, burns

5.  Investigations and results
6.  Drugs administered, time and doses

The communication between the referring and receiving clinicians is a two-way process. The referring doctor describes the injuries and the state of the physiological systems. The receiving doctor accepts the patient and offers advice on management. In addition, the receiving clinician must communicate with the admitting ward area (e.g. neurosurgical ICU) to check on the bed state before accepting a new patient, except in clearly defined circumstances where the urgency of surgical intervention overrides the availability of a postoperative bed. The latter situation is rare, but must be recognised immediately in order to avoid delay. This is aided by a formal policy distributed by the neurosurgical unit to the emergency departments and ICUs in the surrounding hospitals (Box 12.10). The policy is of particular importance in acute extradural haematomas following injury, but may also be applied to other operable conditions, such as acute hydrocephalus and some cases of spontaneous intracerebral haemorrhage, providing that the severity, urgency, and operability fit the criteria as described.

Most head injury transfers are in the *intensive* category, requiring intensive care training to specialist registrar level in the medical escort and critical care experience in the trained nurse escort. Patients with an acute extradural haematoma and a deteriorating conscious level have particular urgency. They remain in the intensive category, but must be transferred expeditiously to prevent secondary brain insults. The

---

**Box 12.10.  Life threatening intracranial space occupying lesions**

*Recommendations for the Interhospital Transfer Policy*

In the following life threatening circumstances, the consultant neurosurgeons should be empowered to accept an emergency transfer from those hospitals in the Transfer Group for which the neurosurgical service is specifically responsible, even if there is no available intensive care bed in the hospital, provided that an appropriately staffed and equipped operating theatre can be made available for emergency neurosurgical intervention.

Acute life threatening intracranial space occupying lesions:

- which are predicted to deteriorate rapidly with a high risk of death or disability unless treated surgically without delay
- which are judged to be sufficiently urgent to transfer straight to the operating theatre for life saving surgery before admission to a ward
- in which a favourable outcome is potentially achievable with prompt surgical treatment.

In all other circumstances, the availability of an intensive care bed must be established before accepting a transfer from another hospital with a neurosurgical emergency likely to need intensive care.

If the outcome is considered to be so poor that transfer for acute neurosurgical intervention is futile, the consultant neurosurgeon should be empowered to refuse the patient, irrespective of bed availability. Advice on continuing or withdrawing care should still be provided to the referring clinician.

response time demanded of the transferring ambulance can then legitimately be shortened from the usual 20 minutes to 8 minutes, the same as demanded of a *critical* case. Arranging the ambulance with such urgency requires that the other aspects of care have been addressed and that the medical and nursing escorts are already well briefed and prepared. Otherwise, the ambulance crew will be frustrated by the delay they witness when they arrive, expecting urgent transfer.

To be ready to transfer the patient out within a few minutes of the CT scan confirmation of the extradural haematoma requires slick teamwork during the initial resuscitation. Taking the patient to the scanner constitutes intrahospital transfer, for which stabilisation on a transport ventilator is required. In this way, the team must already be prepared for transport at this stage. It goes without saying that the escorts should be involved in the assessment and resuscitation of the patient as soon as possible. Ideally, they should form part of the trauma team and be called at the outset. They should certainly not be called after the diagnosis has been made and then pressurised to set off with a patient with whom they are unfamiliar.

If the patient presents with evidence of a life threatening head injury, the CT scan should be ordered as early as possible, generally at the end of the primary survey. The team then has the radiographer call-in and CT scan warm-up time in which to complete the secondary survey and resuscitation. Some of the planned plain radiographs (e.g. for minor limb injuries or to clear the thoracolumbar spine) may not have been completed by the time the CT scanner is ready. These can often be deferred in the presence of a life threatening intracranial haemorrhage, sometimes until after transfer to the neurosurgical unit. On the other hand, intraperitoneal bleeding, which itself can compromise the neurological outcome by reducing cerebral perfusion pressure, must be discovered and treated before transfer.

Patients with an isolated, depressed skull fracture, a normal conscious level and no evidence of cerebral contusion or intracranial haemorrhage on the CT scan will be categorised as *ill and unstable* or *ill and stable*. If there is any doubt about the patient's condition, it is unwise to undertake the transfer as ill and stable, without an advanced life support practitioner, so soon after a serious head injury. Referring to Figure 5.1, it can be seen that the presence of an advanced life support practitioner is a key distinction between ill and unstable and ill and stable. Using Figure 5.1 to categorise the patient will help to ensure that resources are allocated appropriately.

Whenever a transfer is agreed for emergency neurosurgical intervention without a guaranteed intensive care bed, the responsible manager should be informed immediately, work with consultants to facilitate arrangements for providing a suitable bed postoperatively and contribute to the audit of the individual case.

If a patient is transferred for emergency neurosurgical intervention without a guaranteed intensive care bed and still requires an intensive care bed postoperatively, the following options should be considered:

- admission into a neurointensive care bed, if one has by then become available
- transferring the patient out into the nearest available neurosurgical intensive care bed
- if the patient is too unstable for transfer, transferring out another, more stable intensive care patient into the nearest appropriate intensive care bed.

## Preparation and packaging

To help prevent hypoxia and hypotension, the tracheal tube and the intravenous lines must be secure. The ICP will increase if there is impaired venous drainage from the brain, which may result from:

- the use of tapes tied around the patient's neck to secure the tracheal tube or a badly applied hard collar, pressing on the jugular veins

- safety straps applied across the thorax for transfer, restricting chest expansion and increasing intrathoracic pressure.

The latter may also decrease venous return, which in turn will reduce cardiac output and may compromise cerebral perfusion.

During transportation, patients will become hypothermic unless significant efforts are made to prevent it. Although mild hypothermia under controlled conditions may help lower ICP and improve outcome in certain groups of patients, hypothermia is associated with an increase in mortality in the patient with multiple injuries. At low temperatures, platelet dysfunction and a progressive coagulopathy develop. Hypothermia is associated with a greater risk of infection. At the other extreme, hyperthermia is also a risk factor in head injured patients, though it is rarely evident within the first 24 hours after the primary insult. All patients transferred with severe head injuries should have their core temperature monitored with the aim of maintaining normothermia.

## Transportation

Ideally all patients should be resuscitated on a trolley which can be used for any subsequent transfer. For transfers within the hospital, staying on an emergency trolley throughout resuscitation and transfer is feasible and avoids unnecessary movement with its risks of discomfort, further injury or dislodgement of tubes and lines. Transferring to another hospital usually demands a change of trolley, as ambulance trolleys tend to be too narrow for optimum care in the resuscitation room.

Loading a severely head injured patient into an ambulance or other transport vehicle can cause significant problems due to the inherent instability of both the cardiovascular system and the cerebral circulation. A head-down position can cause rises in ICP and should be avoided, except momentarily (in the emergency department or ICU) to insert a central venous line, if indicated. A head-up position is recommended, but care should be taken to avoid hypotension associated with venous pooling in the legs. The aim should be to keep the patient 10° head up whenever possible.

Every effort should be made to minimise the cardiovascular effects of acceleration, deceleration, and cornering by travelling as smoothly as possible at a moderately constant speed. The patient is generally placed head first into a land ambulance, allowing access to the head by the crew. Sudden braking then mimics a head-down position. In a helicopter, the patient is normally loaded head first, but as the aircraft tilts nose down to make good forward speed, the patient is again head down.

En route, observations of the oxygen saturation, end-tidal $CO_2$, pulse, and blood pressure should be noted every 5–10 minutes, the same frequency with which these observations are made on an anaesthetised patient in the operating theatre. A dedicated chart should be available in all critical care areas from which transfers are likely to take place. An example of such a chart is shown in Figure 12.3. The chart serves as an *aide memoire* for the handover at the receiving hospital and a copy can be stored for subsequent analysis and audit.

| ICU TRANSFER FORM<br>INSTRUCTIONS FOR USE OF THIS FORM<br>To be used for all patients transferred to ICU – this is a legal record of transfer | | Time | | | | | | | | | | | |
|---|---|---|---|---|---|---|---|---|---|---|---|---|---|
| | | Drugs | | | | | | | | | | | |
| **PATIENT DETAILS** | **TRANSFER DETAILS** | Monitoring<br>SaO$_2$<br>ETCO$_2$ | | | | | | | | | | | |
| | | 220 | | | | | | | | | | | |
| | | 200 | | | | | | | | | | | |
| Audit data: | | 180 | | | | | | | | | | | |
| | | 160 | | | | | | | | | | | |
| | | 140 | | | | | | | | | | | |
| | | 120.... | | | | | | | | | | | |
| **HISTORY & CLINICAL FINDINGS** | | Fluids | | | | | | | | | | | |
| | | Please list any precautions taken for fractured spine at any level | | | | | | | | | | | |
| **STABILISATION TIME** | **AMBULANCE DETAILS** | TRANSFER COMMENTS/PROBLEMS: | | | | | | | | | | | |
| **STAFF ARRANGING TRANSFER** | **ESCORTING PERSONNEL** | | | | | | | | | | | | |
| At transferring hospital | Doctor | COMMENTS OF RECEIVING DOCTOR: | | | | | | | | | | | |
| At recipient hospital | Nurse/ODA | | | | | | | | | | | | |
| **VENTILATION DURING TRANSFER** | **MONITORING** | Signature of receiving doctor: | | | | | | | | | | | |

**Figure 12.3.** Critical care transfer record.

**Summary**

Special situations require the transfer team to think beyond the generic use of the ACCEPT system and apply it to particular problems. Patients fall into three groups – trauma, medical, and paediatric. Pathological processes can then be considered within each separate body region or physiological system and incorporated into the ACCEPT system.

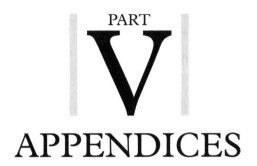

PART

# V

# APPENDICES

# A

# Legal issues and documentation

**Objectives**

- Understand legal issues surrounding transfers and retrievals.
- Understand the importance of transfer documentation.

The word "negligence" is often used when discussing legal issues. It is therefore of some importance to outline what it means. In order to bring a case of negligence the following criteria have to be fulfilled.

- A duty of care must be established.
- The failure of that duty of care must be established.
- The victim must have suffered some damage.
- There must be a chain of causation which links all three of the above.

Unless all the above criteria are established, and especially the chain of causation, negligence cannot be proved.

In the United Kingdom the health service in general and each provider unit in particular has a duty of care to provide intensive care treatment for its patients. It therefore may not be long before a patient sues for damages caused by the failure to provide adequate specialist treatment in respect of intensive care facilities, thus necessitating the transfer and putting the patient at risk.

## BOUNDARIES OF CLINICAL RESPONSIBILITIES

The consultant in charge of the patient's care remains in charge until the patient has been assessed, by the clinician who will undertake the transfer of that patient, and agrees to undertake the transfer. After this, the responsibility for clinical care ultimately rests with the consultant in charge of the team or person undertaking the transfer.

This responsibility will remain until the patient has been handed over and accepted by the team at the receiving hospital. Negligence claims in respect of morbidity and

119

mortality have to prove the likely origin (time and place) of the act or omission which resulted in injury in order to apportion blame correctly. In other words a receiving hospital cannot be held responsible for an act or omission which occurred before they accepted responsibility.

The boundaries of clinical responsibility become blurred when dealing with specialist referrals. For instance, a referring hospital may receive advice from the specialist centre who may indicate a course of treatment to be started prior to transfer. The question arises who is responsible for the care of the patient prior to transfer; is it the referring medical team or is it the receiving specialist medical team who are offering advice? A simple example may be a head injured patient in one hospital being referred to a neurosciences centre at another hospital; the neurosciences hospital recommend 500 ml of 20% mannitol, the referring hospital decline to administer this drug, and there is a subsequent legal argument as to who was responsible for the poor outcome of the patient.

# PROFESSIONAL LIABILITY/ACCOUNTABILITY

In the United Kingdom employees of NHS trusts who are acting on behalf of that trust, whether on the hospital premises or as agents of the hospital in transferring patients or indeed acting as members of the hospital care teams, are indemnified by that trust. Some medical teams who undertake retrieval/repatriation work in which they will be caring for patients transferred between remote units have to have special dispensation from their employers before the liability for this work is accepted.

# DISABILITY AND DISABLEMENT ENTITLEMENT/INSURANCE COVER

All NHS staff are entitled to benefit from the NHS benefits scheme. This scheme is separate from the NHS pension scheme and provides a spectrum of benefits to the employee in relation to temporary or permanent inability to work up to and including death. In essence, the benefits are based on the present salary of the employee, years of service and, in the case of death, any dependants. These benefits are subject to a form of means test and may be curtailed if other benefits from other sources are being paid out.

Currently all NHS trusts are required to sign up to employer's liability. At present details of benefits which may be obtained from this scheme are sketchy; what seems to be clear is that some form of negligence on the part of the employer has to be proved.

An increasing number of trusts are taking out personal accident insurance schemes in order to provide some form of cover for injury or death following an accident whilst on trust business outside the hospital. Many of the schemes are based around the payout of £250 000 per employee. There is widespread concern that this level of benefit may not be sufficient for cover of the long term needs of a permanently disabled trust employee or his or her family in the event of the employee's death. Much work is currently being undertaken to identify the appropriate level of accident insurance required.

# DOCUMENTATION

The decision to transfer and the act of transferring a critically ill patient from one hospital to another, and even within a hospital, requires the agreement and cooperation of a number of people.

In addition, the fact that a critically ill patient is to be exposed to a hostile environment during the transfer increases the likelihood of morbidity or even peri-transfer mortality due to adverse incidents.

In many instances there are no problems during transfer; however, when problems do arise, poor documentation will make it difficult to investigate. Only when problems have arisen and questions are asked do we realise the inadequacy of our documentation.

## Who will ask the questions?

*The consumer*

The public are increasingly aware of their rights to be informed of the care given to themselves and their relatives. The medical and nursing professions are being held increasingly accountable. The public *will* ask questions and expect clear answers.

*Our peers*

Clinical governance embraces the concept of adverse event recording. Therefore we are encouraged to record and investigate adverse incidents using clinical incident systems. The transfer of critically ill patients is likely to generate a significant number of adverse incidents.

*The litigious*

The transfer of critically ill patients is likely to generate a number of adverse incidents – some of these may be of great interest to those involved in medical negligence work.

## Questions and answers

Knowing the likely questions will better enable practitioners to ensure that the information required to enable them to provide a reasonable explanation is available in the medical notes.

It is traditional to record events in the hospital notes in chronological order and, where possible, contemporaneously.

A simple framework for "what to document" might be:

| | |
|---|---|
| **Why** is the patient being transferred? | What has happened to the patient? What treatment is needed? What resources are required? |
| **Who** has been informed? | Communication with relatives and all those clinically responsible |
| **What** might happen in transfer? | Proof of risk assessment and proper stabilisation |

Because notes are written chronologically, there will inevitably be several sets of documentation covering:

- the referring hospital
- the transfer itself
- the receiving hospital.

It is essential that the documentation reads as one continuous record. The referring hospital notes should clearly summarise:

- the patient's history
- the reasons for transfer
- who has been involved in the negotiations
- the assessments of the risks of transfer
- the consequent stabilisation procedures
- ending up with a statement: "patient transferred to ★★★★★ hospital".

## Hospital notes

Hospital notes are a legal record, a log of events. They should record the clinical information which leads to the reasoning behind the medical treatment. Doctors' handwriting is notorious for its illegibility and there seems little point in using the pen to communicate, when no one else can decipher what is written. In general if a fact or event is not documented then, in law, it has not happened. If an entry is illegible, then it is not only failing to communicate but could be ruled as inadmissible.

As with all documentation, each entry in hospital notes must be dated, timed and the author's name and contact details clearly appended. It is also good practice to note the location of the patient. For example:

*23/11/2002 12:23 Theatre 4 Smith J. (SHO Anaesthesia) bleep 2341*

It is always important to indicate the date and time when events occurred as well as the time the entry was made. This is especially important when dealing with transfers, as the chronology of events and discussions may be crucial in an enquiry.

If the pace of events and circumstances dictate that some entries must be made at a later time, then this must be made clear; the notes should state that it is a non-contemporaneous entry and include the time of the event referred to as well as the time the entry was made.

## Transfer record

To cover the actual transfer period it would seem good practice to use some form of transfer documentation, which summarises some of the above and details the care given during the transfer. Just as both hospitals will have a unique record number for each patient, the ambulance service will issue a unique record number for each ambulance journey – the incident number. This number should be recorded on the transfer form to facilitate audit and investigation of adverse incidents.

Copies of the transfer form should be filed in the referring hospital's notes, the receiving hospital's notes and a central point for audit.

## The handover

It is not uncommon for the medical or surgical teams to ask the anaesthetic service to manage a transfer; it should be made clear in the notes that those involved in the transfer have received a detailed handover. The handover is important as it would seem that by accepting the task of transferring the patient, the anaesthetist, and therefore the consultant on call, has accepted the responsibility for that patient until he is handed over to the care of the team at the receiving hospital, where it is normally implicit that this team then assumes clinical responsibility.

**Summary**

- Effective oral and written communication is an essential part of the transfer process.
- Oral communication must be structured, clear, and concise.
- The documentation of the events surrounding a transfer is important not only for clinical audit, but also as a defence against potential litigation.
- The last page of the referring hospital's notes, the transfer form, and the first pages of the receiving hospital's notes should read as a seamless progression of events. The reader should be able to follow the thought processes and the chain of events which brought about and completed the successful transfer of the most critically ill patient, and the notes should reflect the high standard of care and communication during this difficult time.

# APPENDIX

# B

# Safety

---

**Objectives**

- Consider safety issues within transfers and retrievals.

---

## SAFETY FOR THE CARER

All life support training programmes emphasise the importance of ensuring that the carer is safe. An injured carer is of no use to the patient and can be a hazard to the rest of the team.

### Universal precautions

The use of gloves and, where appropriate, safety spectacles or goggles is to be encouraged. All waste (especially sharps) should be appropriately disposed of.

### Moving and handling

It is a requirement that all staff should receive moving and handling training. Medical staff are not excluded. The use of devices such as Patslides has significantly reduced the need for any form of lifting. However, currently it is inevitable that the transport stretcher will have to be lifted into the ambulance or aircraft and staff should be aware of this when loading up the stretcher with heavy items such as monitors and oxygen cylinders.

### Clothing and footwear

Warm clothing and substantial footwear are mandatory. Weather conditions may change significantly en route. Theatre clogs are entirely inappropriate for entering and exiting ambulances.

## Inside the vehicle

The ambulance crew are responsible for the general safety of the patient and the accompanying staff; it is therefore important that members of the transferring team listen to the advice of the ambulance crew. On entering the vehicle, staff should familiarise themselves with the general layout of the interior, making special note of features such as grab rails. In general, if the patient is well resuscitated and has been stabilised prior to transfer the accompanying team must remain seated during the journey. Seat belts must be used. If it becomes necessary to leave the seat then the driver should be alerted. The vehicle should be stopped; however, if this is not possible, then the "kneeling tripod position" (see Figure B.1) may offer some stability.

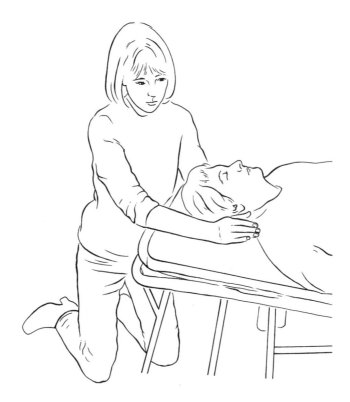

**Figure B.1.**   Kneeling tripod position

# SAFETY FOR THE PATIENT

A full assessment of the patient must be made by those responsible for the care of that patient in transit. A full handover from the medical team responsible for the care of the patient up to the point of transfer is required in order to assess:

- what is wrong with the patient
- what resuscitation is needed to stabilise the patient
- what can go wrong during the transfer.

The packaging of the patient must be undertaken bearing in mind that the transfer environment is hostile. The patient is at risk of:

- exposure
- inertial forces.

Despite the fact that modern ambulances have efficient heating systems it is not uncommon for patients to be exposed to thermal changes during the transfer and this usually results in heat loss.

Inertial forces may adversely affect the physiology of the patient. Although the patient may not be exposed to G forces anywhere near those experienced by military pilots, the critically ill patient is often intolerant of inertial forces experienced in an ambulance. This is especially the case if they are volume depleted. Inertial forces can cause dislodgement of vital equipment which must be secured correctly and constantly checked. The endotracheal tube, drains, and venous cannulae are particularly vulnerable to dislodgement by movement.

## Timeliness

There is often a sense of urgency during the organisation and execution of a transfer. The team should remember that in nearly every instance a proper assessment and stabilisation does take time and, if correctly undertaken, should lead to the transfer of a stable patient.

Once inside the vehicle, the escorting medical staff should dictate the approximate speed of the vehicle. Providing the patient has been resuscitated and stabilised there should be no requirement for excessive speed. High velocities will increase the likelihood of excessive inertial forces in association with sudden deceleration and rotational forces when going round corners.

It is important to ensure that there is agreement as to the exact location of the receiving hospital and within that hospital the intensive care unit. The best access route for the receiving unit should also be clarified.

**Summary**

The safety of both staff and patients should be assured. This is done by appropriate and adequate risk assessment and attention to detail.

# C

# Helicopter transfers

Transfer of patients by air and in particular by helicopter has advantages in sparsely populated areas or a maritime environment. A helicopter can deliver medical, nursing or paramedical expertise to enable resuscitation to proceed. It can take part in the retrieval exercise or can assist with a road based retrieval. However, in a solely urban environment, helicopters may have no advantage over a well equipped road based service.

Helicopters are frequently small and provide only limited access to the patient. Ambient light may be limited. Noise and vibration can make monitoring the patient difficult. It may also be difficult to secure or adjust equipment. The range of the aircraft may be relatively short. Landing places are limited, requiring extra transfers by road vehicle at the beginning and end of the journey. Consequently there may be little advantage in terms of journey time if the distance to be travelled is short. The cost of transfer by helicopter is also high.

Road vehicles are, in contrast, cheaper to deploy and are manned by personnel who are familiar to medical and nursing staff. They are frequently well equipped although standards vary locally and regionally.

## A – ASSESS PATIENT AND SITUATION

The job of the helicopter crew is to provide facilities for transfer. They may have knowledge of basic life support and care of patients in a military setting. They cannot be expected to provide medical or nursing care during transfer. They will require details of the patient's name, home address and current location, exact destination, and the length of the journey. In addition, they will need details of diagnosis, condition and stability, treatment completed or in progress, level of support, and monitoring. They may wish to discuss the feasibility of undertaking the entire journey by air and the location of liaison points with road ambulance services if these are required.

## C – CONTROL OF THE SITUATION

The helicopter aircrew are in control of the aircraft and are responsible for the safety of the craft and its occupants. Their instructions must be obeyed. It is their decision whether to undertake the transfer. The patient must be in as stable and safe a condition as possible. Primary survey and resuscitation should proceed along advanced life support guidelines with particular attention paid to securing the airway by tracheal intubation and ventilation if necessary. The risk of pneumothorax should be assessed. Intravenous access must be secured and fluids and medications commenced prior to transfer. A semi-rigid collar must be applied to the neck and the patient transferred on a stretcher which affords protection to the axial skeleton.

# C – COMMUNICATION

Communication from aircraft is by radio. Operational frequencies allow communication between aircraft and civil and military airfields. It is unlikely that the aircrew will be able to communicate directly with a land based ambulance or its control centre or a hospital switchboard or an emergency department. Communications are usually relayed and must therefore be clear and concise. A working knowledge of the phonetic alphabet and voice procedure is useful (see Chapter 9).

Noise levels inside helicopters may make normal speech incomprehensible unless the communicants are face to face. Hence the command "watch my lips". It is usual for medical attendants to be issued with headphones which will enhance verbal communication between themselves and the aircrew. However, medical attendants are commonly switched out of communications between aircrew and their land base.

The use of headphones and the noisy environment may render alarms on medical equipment inaudible. Equipment with visible alarm systems should be used if possible.

Lines of communication should be established between those retrieving or despatching the patient and medical staff at the destination, providing a succinct systematic summary of the situation. This must include identification of the personnel undertaking the transfer, basic details of the patient, a brief description of the problem, treatment undertaken and that which may be required on arrival. Named individuals and telephone numbers should be identified for liaison.

# E – EVALUATE

Transfer of a critically ill patient must be undertaken only if it is associated with the provision of improved medical care and the possibility of improved outcome. Usually the requirement for transfer is self-evident. However, there is evidence which suggests that many transfers do not fulfil these criteria and that serious physiological destabilisation may occur during transfer, to the possible detriment of the patient. Transfer by air may not shorten the duration of the journey if land based vehicles must be used at each end.

> The decision to transfer by air rather than road should be given careful consideration.

# P – PREPARATION AND PACKAGING

The environment inside a helicopter has some unusual features. Ambient light is poor. The noise level is high. Unless the aircraft has been designed for the transfer of patients there may be no purpose built anchorage points for a stretcher. Vibration may interfere with the function of intravenous infusion controllers if they rely on drop counters. It may also be difficult to keep the patient warm without extra insulation from cold and draughts.

Monitoring and therapeutic equipment should be small and compact, easily securable, and visible. A case or other stowage bag should be taken to pack equipment for the return journey. Equipment should be known to function in such an environment and should not emit any signal that could interfere with navigational or other onboard electrical systems. Ventilatory, intravenous, and other equipment must be adequately secured to the patient because the confined space and environmental considerations will make replacement difficult, if not impossible. All necessary drugs and equipment should be carried in an appropriately designed pack for ease of identification, preparation, and use.

The patient must be in a stable physiological condition before undertaking the transfer. Particular attention should be paid to ventilatory and circulatory status. Access to the patient may be difficult in the confined environment with little opportunity to make major therapeutic adjustments. Tracheal intubation and ventilation is the safest option and should be mandatory if the patient's GCS is $\leqslant 9$. Chest drains should be inserted if there is a risk of pneumothorax. Hypoxaemia may occur at high altitudes because the fall in atmospheric $PO_2$ will lead to a reduction in alveolar oxygen. The reduction in atmospheric pressure at altitude will increase the volume of gas filled cavities which include pneumothoraces, the stomach and bowel and the cranium and brain if there are fractures through the frontal or maxillary sinuses or the ethmoid plate. Tracheal tube cuffs should be inflated with saline. The patient must be transferred on a stretcher which affords protection to the axial skeleton. This should also be firmly secured to the helicopter with CAA approved fastenings.

> For specialised transport, e.g. helicopters, head, ear and eye protection will be required for both the patient and the team.

Accompanying personnel must be suitably attired in protective clothing. Personal equipment to be carried should include a mobile telephone with a directory of useful numbers, money and credit cards, driver's licence, relevant map, and a snack. Transport back to base for personnel and equipment should be organised before the transfer is undertaken. Motion or air sickness may influence the choice of personnel. Nonsedating prophylaxis in the form of medications such as Cinnarizine should be instituted at a suitable interval prior to departure.

## T – TRANSPORTATION

Few hospitals are equipped with a helicopter landing area immediately outside their doors. It is therefore usual for patients requiring transfer by air to be taken to the aircraft by road vehicle and delivered to hospital at their destination in the same way. Thus during transfer the patient will be moved to a new location several times. Transfer of location is associated with physiological destabilisation and disconnection of equipment and should be undertaken with care.

## SAFETY CONSIDERATIONS

When patients are transferred by air (helicopter or fixed wing), special precautions are needed.

The pilot is in overall charge of safety on board. His prime responsibility is the safety of the aircraft. Staff should not approach the aircraft unless the pilot indicates that it is safe to do so (usually by showing the thumbs up sign).

Always approach the aircraft from the front and in clear vision of the pilots who will direct you.

Most people will recognise the potential danger of propellor blades in a fixed wing aircraft but will fail to recognise the danger of the tail rotor in a helicopter.

**Never go around the back of a helicopter!**

Moving helicopter rotor blades, which are usually invisible, can cause significant downdraft of the order of 10 tons. This can cause a great deal of flying debris and can even blow the unwary over. Remember that the blades are only fully horizontal when at full speed and at slower speeds they dip down towards the tips.

Within the aircraft the general safety rules for ambulances apply but the environment is even less friendly due to:

- noise
- vibration
- lighting
- cramped conditions.

**Summary**

Helicopter transfers have a particular place and particular problems. They should only be undertaken when there is clear benefit to the patient. Staff undertaking such transfers should use appropriate equipment and be adequately trained.

# INDEX